What Rocket's immune system doesn't "know" can't hurt him.

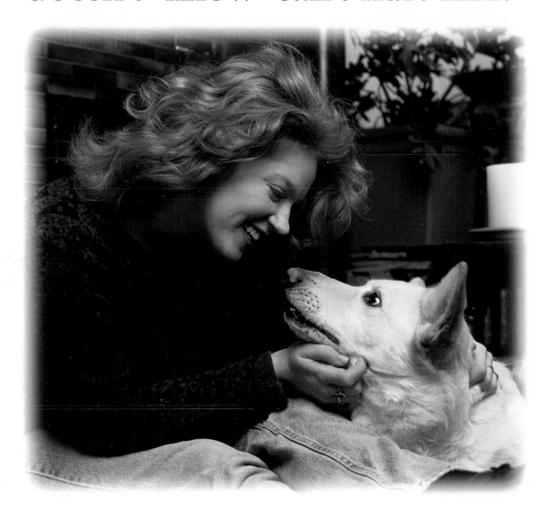

Not novel protein. _Modified_ protein.

At Purina® we're committed to improving the lives of pets and their owners through nutrition. Research into the mechanisms of food allergy is just one example. We understand that by reducing a protein's molecular weight it becomes less antigenic. So instead of focusing on novel protein, we modified a protein to minimize the immune system's adverse response. Purina applied this knowledge to **CNM® HA-Formula®** Diet. The first truly hypoallergenic diet. So dogs like R Because when he feels better, we all do.

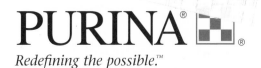

D1206597

PURINA®
Redefining the possible.™

Published by The Gloyd Group, Inc.
Wilmington, Delaware
© 1999 by Ralston Purina Company.
All rights reserved.
Printed in the United States of America.
Ralston Purina Company: Checkerboard Square, Saint Louis, Missouri, 63188
First printing, 1999.

ISBN 0-9678005-0-1

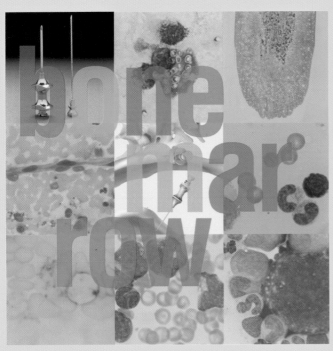

Bone Marrow Evaluation in Dogs and Cats

Maxey L. Wellman, DVM, PhD, DACVP
M. Judith Radin, DVM, PhD, DACVP

Ralston Purina Company
Clinical Handbook Series

Table of Contents

Introduction

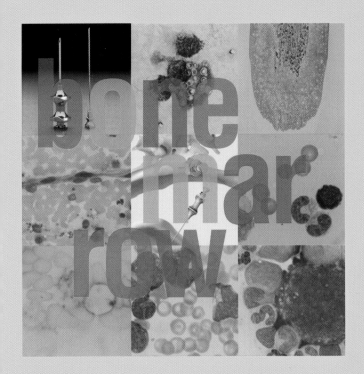

The bone marrow is the major site for hematopoiesis in the healthy adult animal. At birth and during early postnatal life, hematopoiesis occurs in the marrow of all bones. With maturity, active hematopoiesis is restricted to the axial skeleton (flat bones, such as the pelvis, ribs, sternum, and skull) and ends of the long bones. In times of increased demand for production of blood cells, hematopoiesis can expand within the long bones and into extramedullary sites, such as the spleen, liver, and lymph nodes. Hematopoietic tissue in the bone marrow is composed of progenitor cells capable of producing granulocytes, monocytes/macrophages, erythrocytes, lymphocytes, and platelets.

In addition, stromal cells, such as adipocytes, fibroblasts, macrophages, and endothelial cells, play a key role in providing a stable supporting structure for the hematopoietic progenitor cells as well as necessary growth factors to sustain hematopoiesis. An understanding of normal hematopoiesis is helpful in interpreting bone marrow aspirates from dogs and cats that are ill. Abnormalities in the bone marrow may be reflected in changes observed in the peripheral blood. For proper interpretation of a bone marrow aspirate, it is essential to perform a concurrent complete blood count (CBC or hemogram).

This book, **Bone Marrow Evaluation in Dogs and Cats**, is divided into 3 parts: **Part I** covers basic information on cellular development as well as when and how to perform bone marrow evaluations and how to interpret the results. **Part II** expands on the basic information of Part I with discussions on abnormal bone marrow, including neoplasias, and a chapter devoted to case studies. Reference material is found in **Part III**.

Part I

Chapter 1: Normal Hematopoiesis

Hematopoiesis is the process by which terminally differentiated blood cells develop from undifferentiated stem cells. All hematopoietic cells are derived from a common pluripotential stem cell, which gives rise to both lymphoid and myeloid (nonlymphoid) multipotential stem cells (*Figure 1*). Lymphoid and myeloid stem cells further differentiate into lymphoid and myeloid progenitor cells. Stem cells are characterized by their capacity for self-renewal and their ability to differentiate along multiple cell lineages, whereas progenitor cells have little if any capacity for self-renewal and are committed to cell production along a limited number of lineages. Stem cells morphologically resemble lymphoid cells and are present in such low numbers that they are difficult to recognize in bone marrow aspirates.

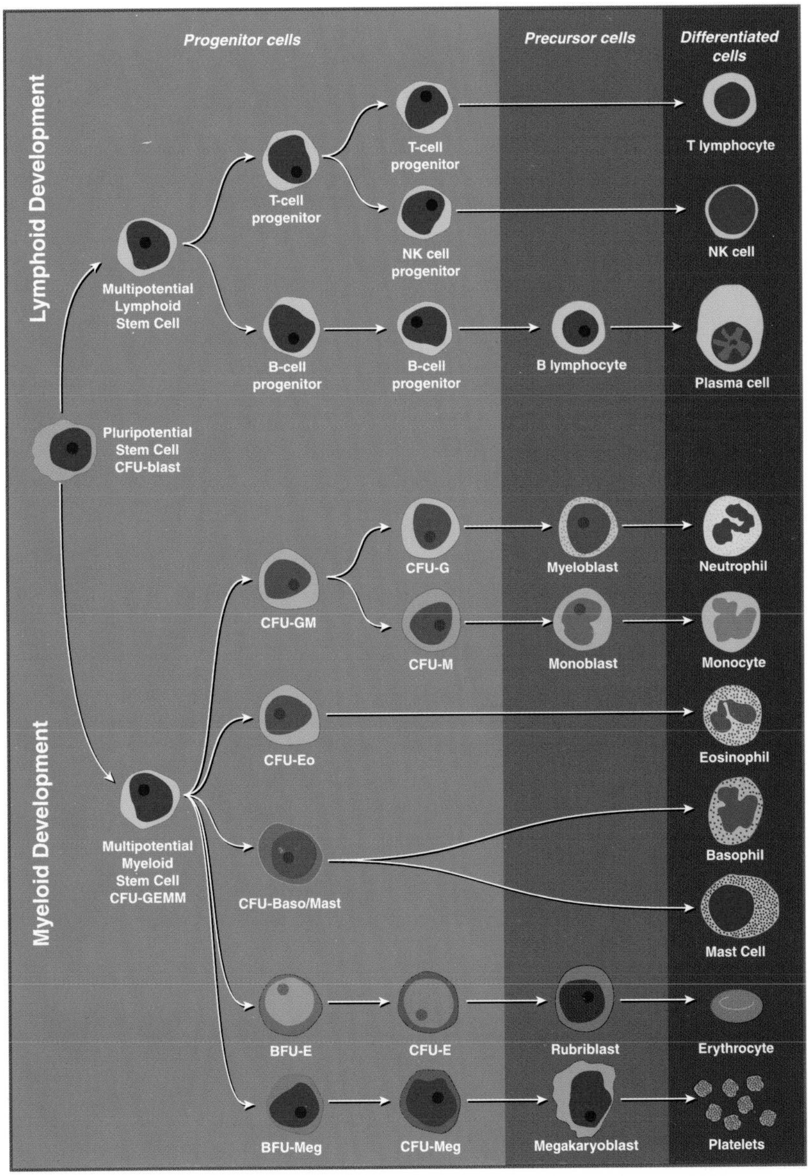

Subsets of committed lymphoid progenitors differentiate into B lymphocyte, T lymphocyte, and natural killer (NK) cell precursors, which undergo further differentiation in the bone marrow, thymus, or peripheral lymphoid tissues. Subsets of committed myeloid progenitor cells differentiate into erythroid, granulocytic, monocytic, and megakaryocytic precursors, which become morphologically recognizable cells of the specific lineage. Terminal differentiation of myeloid precursors results in release of red blood cells (RBCs), granulocytes (neutrophils, eosinophils, and basophils), monocytes, and platelets from the bone marrow into the peripheral blood.

A variety of *in vitro* colony-forming assays have been used to evaluate stem cell and progenitor cell commitment and differentiation. In these assays, bone marrow cells are cultured in semisolid media with various lineage-specific growth factors. These colony-forming assays have provided tremendous insight into mechanisms of normal and abnormal hematopoiesis. Although they are not used very often in clinical veterinary medicine, these tests are helpful in providing an understanding of the hierarchy of colony-forming cells and an appreciation for how abnormalities in stem cells or treatment with cytokines and growth factors may affect multiple cell lines.

The *in vitro* counterpart of the pluripotential hematopoietic stem cell is the colony-forming unit blast (CFU-blast) and the *in vitro* counterpart of committed myeloid progenitor

Figure 1. Differentiation of hematopoietic cells. (Modified from: Cotran RS, Kumar V, Robbins, SL, eds. In: *Pathologic Basis of Disease*. Philadelphia, PA: WB Saunders Co; 1994; 585. Illustration by Tim Vojt.)

cells is the colony-forming unit granulocyte-erythrocyte-monocyte-megakaryocyte (CFU-GEMM). Further commitment of cells from CFU-GEMM results in colony-forming units granulocyte-macrophage (CFU-GM), colony-forming units granulocyte (CFU-G), colony-forming units monocyte/macrophage (CFU-M), colony-forming units eosinophil (CFU-Eo), burst-forming units erythroid (BFU-E), colony-forming units erythroid (CFU-E), burst-forming units megakaryocyte (BFU-Meg), and colony-forming units megakaryocyte (CFU-Meg). The *in vitro* counterpart of basophil progenitors may be related to mast cell progenitors and currently is designated as colony-forming unit basophil/mast cell (CFU-Baso/Mast). Although lymphoid colony-forming units have been recognized, lymphopoiesis involves extramarrow sites for differentiation and maturation of different lymphocyte subsets, especially for T lymphocytes.

Cytokines and Growth Factors

Hematopoiesis is regulated by a variety of cytokines and growth factors, many of which are secreted by cells of the bone marrow microenvironment. These include macrophages, endothelial cells, fibroblasts, and adipocytes. The bone marrow microenvironment also includes the extracellular matrix, which may be critical for binding cytokines to facilitate interaction with hematopoietic cells. Growth factors can act singly or synergistically and their effects on a particular cell type may be concentration dependent. Some growth factors have effects on multiple cell types. The effects of hematopoietic growth factors are mediated by binding to specific receptors and activation of intracellular signaling pathways to promote cell proliferation or maturation. Some of the hematopoietic growth factors and their effects are listed in *Table 1*.

Veterinary medicine has begun to take advantage of the effects of some of these cytokines and growth factors to stimulate hematopoiesis in specific clinical situations. Cytokines have been used therapeutically for diseases of hematopoietic stem cells; to improve host defense in animals with neutropenia, defective neutrophil and macrophage function, and immunodeficiency diseases; and to stimulate hematopoiesis following chemotherapy. However, restricted species activity has been shown for some cytokines, and some dogs and cats develop antibodies against human cytokines. Development of species-specific growth factors and cytokines should alleviate this problem.

Myelopoiesis

Myelopoiesis involves production of granulocytes (neutrophils, eosinophils, basophils) and monocytes. Committed myeloid progenitor cells are stimulated by interleukin-3 (IL-3) and granulocyte/macrophage colony-stimulating factor (GM-CSF) to produce CFU-GM, CFU-Eo, and CFU-Baso/Mast. Multiple cytokines stimulate CFU-GM to differentiate into myeloblasts or monoblasts, which are the morphologically recognizable precursors of neutrophils and monocytes. CFU-Eo differentiate into mature eosinophils, primarily in response to IL-5. CFU-Baso/Mast differentiate into basophils and mast cells, although there is some controversy about whether basophils and mast cells share a common progenitor.

Nuclear and cytoplasmic characteristics are used to classify granulocytic precursors. The cytomorphologic characteristics and sequence of maturation of granulocytic cells are listed in *Table 2*. The most mature feature takes precedence in cell classification. Myeloblasts are characterized by a round nucleus with diffuse, finely stippled chromatin, and a prominent nucleolus. The cytoplasm is relatively basophilic and usually does not contain granules (*Figure 2*). Chromatin becomes progressively more condensed and the cytoplasm becomes progressively less basophilic at each successive stage of maturation. Granule formation, which begins at the progranulocyte stage, and nuclear segmentation, which begins at the metamyelocyte stage, are characteristic features of granulocyte maturation (*Figure 3*). The

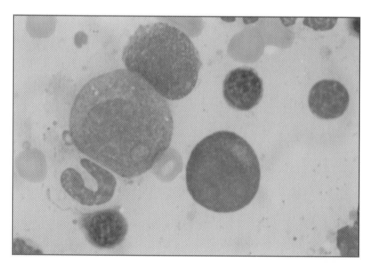

Figure 2. Myeloid and erythroid precursors from the bone marrow of a dog with normal myelopoiesis. A myeloblast is shown in the center left and a rubriblast is shown in the lower right of the field. Myeloblasts usually have lighter staining chromatin and cytoplasm than rubriblasts. Nucleoli are prominent in both the myeloblast and the rubriblast. Wright's stain, 1000X.

Table 1. Selected Hematopoietic Cytokines and Growth Factors

Cytokine/ Growth Factor	Function
Erythropoietin	• Stimulates growth and differentiation of erythroid and megakaryocytic progenitors
Thrombopoietin	• Stimulates production of megakaryocytes and platelets
GM-CSF	• Promotes growth and differentiation of multipotential myeloid progenitor cells • Stimulates production of neutrophils, monocytes, eosinophils, and basophils • Primes phagocytic and chemotactic function of granulocytes and monocytes
G-CSF	• Enhances differentiation and activation of neutrophils
M-CSF	• Induces monocyte/macrophage growth and differentiation • Stimulates phagocytic and secretory function of monocytes/macrophages
IL-1	• Induces expression of multiple cytokines • Synergistic with IL-3 in stimulating proliferation of hematopoietic progenitor cells • Induces synthesis of acute phase reactants
IL-2	• Induces proliferation and activation of T cells, B cells, and NK cells
IL-3	• Synergistic with lineage restricted factors to stimulate production and differentiation of macrophages, neutrophils, eosinophils, and basophils • Supports proliferation of multipotential progenitor cells

Cytokine/ Growth Factor	Function
IL-4	• Diverse effects on T cells, monocytes, and granulocytes • Synergistic with erythropoietin, GM-CSF, and G-CSF
IL-5	• Stimulates growth and differentiation of eosinophils • Chemotactic for eosinophils and activates eosinophil function
IL-6	• Stimulates hematopoietic progenitor cells • Induces maturation of megakaryocytes and increases platelet number • Induces production of acute phase reactants
IL-8	• Chemotactic activity for neutrophils, T cells, and basophils • Activates release of lysosomal enzymes from neutrophils • Induces adhesion of neutrophils to endothelial cells
IL-9	• Synergistic with erythropoietin to support development of erythroid burst-forming units
IL-11	• Synergistic with IL-3 to increase size, number, and ploidy of megakaryocytes
Stem cell factor	• Synergistic with various growth factors to stimulate myeloid, erythroid, and lymphoid progenitors • Stimulates proliferation and maturation of mast cells
TNF-α	• Mediates expression of genes for growth factors and cytokines, transcription factors, receptors, inflammatory mediators, and acute phase proteins resulting in a wide variety of effects

GM-CSF	*Granulocyte/macrophage colony-stimulating factor*
G-CSF	*Granulocyte colony-stimulating factor*
M-CSF	*Macrophage colony-stimulating factor*
IL-1-9, 11	*Interleukins 1 to 9, and 11*
TNF-α	*Tumor necrosis factor alpha*

Modified from: Raskin RE. Myelopoiesis and myeloproliferative disorders. *Vet Clin North Am Small Anim Prac.* September, 1996;1025.

Table 2. Cytomorphologic Features and Sequence of Maturation of Granulocytes in the Bone Marrow

Cell	Cytomorphologic Features	Cell	Cytomorphologic Features
Myeloblast *Figure 2*	• Large size • Round to oval nucleus • Finely stippled chromatin • One or more prominent nucleoli • Moderately basophilic cytoplasm • Type I myeloblasts: agranular cytoplasm • Type II myeloblasts: few (<15) small azurophilic cytoplasmic granules	Metamyelocyte *Figure 3*	• Continued condensation of chromatin • Indented, kidney bean-shaped nucleus • Slightly basophilic cytoplasm in neutrophilic metamyelocyte • Moderately basophilic cytoplasm in eosinophilic and basophilic metamyelocyte • Staining characteristics of specific granules identify cells as neutrophilic, eosinophilic, or basophilic metamyelocytes
Promyelocyte (Progranulocyte) *Figure 3*	• Size similar to myeloblast • Nucleoli usually are absent • Moderately basophilic cytoplasm • Numerous azurophilic (primary) cytoplasmic granules • Absence of specific (secondary) cytoplasmic granules • More cytoplasm and granules than Type II myeloblasts	Band neutrophil *Figure 3*	• Continued condensation of chromatin • Nucleus has parallel sides but may be twisted to form horseshoe or S shape
Myelocyte	• Smaller than a progranulocyte • Some condensation of nuclear chromatin • Few to numerous specific (secondary) granules	Segmented neutrophil (Polymorpho-nuclear leukocyte) *Figure 3*	• Condensed chromatin • Irregular nuclear membrane • Multiple nuclear lobes connected by thin filaments
Neutrophilic myelocyte	• Light blue cytoplasm • Dust-like, faintly pink granules	Eosinophil	• Nucleus may be bilobed • Moderately basophilic cytoplasm • Numerous reddish-orange granules (round in dogs, rod-shaped in cats)
Eosinophilic myelocyte	• Moderately basophilic cytoplasm • Round, reddish-orange granules in dogs • Rod-shaped, reddish-orange granules in cats	Basophil	• Larger than neutrophil • Nucleus may be monocytoid • Moderately basophilic cytoplasm • Few round, metachromatic (dark purple) granules in dogs • Numerous round, pale lavender granules in cats
Basophilic myelocyte	• Metachromatic (dark purple) granules in dogs • Numerous small, round, pinkish granules and fewer large, round, reddish-purple granules in cats		

Modified from: Raskin RE. Myelopoiesis and myeloproliferative disorders. *Vet Clin North Am Small Anim Prac*. September, 1996;1030.

nucleus and cytoplasm usually mature together. Morphologic evidence of asynchronous maturation indicates abnormal hematopoiesis. Compared to erythroid precursors, myeloid cells have less condensed chromatin, less intensely stained cytoplasm, and, depending on the stage of development, have indented or segmented nuclei and cytoplasmic granules (*Figure 4*).

Granulocytic cells sometimes are considered as 2 pools of cells within the bone marrow. Myeloblasts, progranulocytes, and myelocytes are part of the proliferating pool. These cells are capable of division. Metamyelocytes, bands, and cells with segmented nuclei are part of the maturation and storage pool. These cells are no longer capable of division. The number of cells in the storage pool sometimes is used to evaluate the granulocyte reserve in the bone marrow in animals with inflammatory disease. If the storage pool is

Table 3 . Cytomorphologic Features and Sequence of Maturation of Erythroid Cells in the Bone Marrow

Cell	Cytomorphologic Features	Cell	Cytomorphologic Features
Rubriblast *Figure 2*	• Large, round cell • Large, round nucleus • Central or eccentric nucleus • Finely stippled chromatin • Nucleoli or nucleolar rings • Narrow rim of deeply basophilic cytoplasm	Polychro- matophilic rubricyte *Figure 5*	• Continued condensation of nuclear chromatin • Light blue or gray cytoplasm due to synthesis of hemoglobin
		Normochromic rubricyte	• Condensed nuclear chromatin • Cytoplasm stains color of mature erythrocyte
Prorubricyte *Figure 6*	• Similar to rubriblast • Minimal chromatin condensation • Absence of nucleoli or nucleolar rings	Metarubricyte *Figure 6*	• Pyknotic nucleus • Nucleus may be fragmented or partially extruded • Cytoplasm is polychromatophilic or normochromic
Basophilic rubricyte *Figure 5*	• Smaller than prorubricyte • Condensed nuclear chromatin • Narrow rim of deeply basophilic cytoplasm	Erythrocyte *Figure 6*	• Non-nucleated • Tinctorial quality depends on extent of hemoglobin present

Modified from: Raskin RE. Myelopoiesis and myeloproliferative disorders. *Vet Clin North Am Small Anim Prac.* September, 1996;1030.

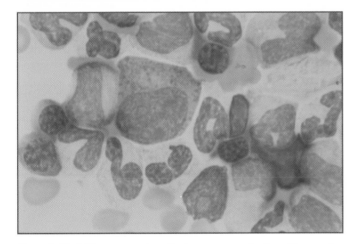

Figure 3. Myeloid precursors from the bone marrow of a dog with normal myelopoiesis. The largest cell is a progranulocyte, which has primary granules in the cytoplasm. Other myeloid precursors include a metamyelocyte, several banded neutrophils, and 2 segmented neutrophils. There also are several rubricytes present. Wright's stain, 1000X.

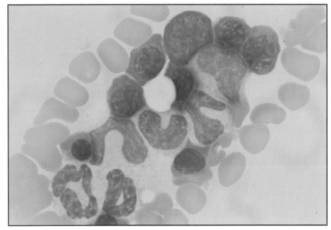

Figure 4. Myeloid and erythroid precursors from the bone marrow of a dog with normal myelopoiesis. Myeloid precursors have less intensely stained chromatin and cytoplasm than erythroid precursors. At later stages of development, myeloid precursors are characterized by nuclear indentation and segmentation and the presence of cytoplasmic granules. The secondary granules often are difficult to visualize in neutrophils from dogs and cats. Erythroid precursors have round nuclei and agranular cytoplasm at all stages of development. Wright's stain, 1000X.

decreased, it may reflect an inability of myelopoiesis to meet peripheral demand, and this may carry a worse prognosis than if the storage pool is adequate.

Monocytes are produced in the bone marrow from monoblasts and promonocytes, but usually very few of these cells are present in normal bone marrow. Further differentiation of monocytes to macrophages occurs in tissues.

Erythropoiesis

Burst-forming units erythroid (BFU-E) are the most immature erythroid cells recognized by *in vitro* colony-forming assays. BFU-E are stimulated by IL-3, IL-4, IL-9, stem cell factor (SCF), and GM-CSF. These cytokines act synergistically with erythropoietin (Epo), which is a hormone produced mainly by peritubular interstitial cells of the kidney. Epo production is enhanced by conditions of renal tissue hypoxia. Although BFU-E respond to Epo, its primary effect is on CFU-E, which differentiate into rubriblasts. Rubriblasts are the earliest morphologically recognizable erythroid lineage cells in routine bone marrow aspirates. Subsequent division and differentiation of erythroid precursors results in prorubricytes, rubricytes, and metarubricytes. The cytomorphologic features and sequence of maturation of cells of the erythroid series are listed in *Table 3*.

Erythropoiesis occurs in erythroblastic islands in which a central macrophage (nurse cell) is surrounded by developing erythroid cells. These islands are easily disrupted during aspiration so are rarely seen on bone marrow smears. As erythroid cells mature, they migrate away from the macrophage toward the abluminal side of the sinusoidal endothelial cells.

Rubriblasts are large, round cells with finely stippled chromatin, nucleoli, and deeply basophilic agranular cyto-plasm (*Figure 2*). As erythroid precursors mature, the chromatin becomes progressively more condensed, the cytoplasm becomes less basophilic, and the cells become smaller (*Figure 5*). At similar stages, the chromatin appears more condensed (darker), and the cytoplasm appears more basophilic in erythroid precursors than in granulocyte precursors. Erythroid precursors also have round nuclei throughout their maturation and are devoid of cytoplasmic granules.

Prorubricytes appear similar to rubriblasts but usually lack nucleoli (*Figure 6*). Rubricytes have more condensed chromatin and are smaller than prorubricytes. Rubricytes with relatively basophilic cytoplasm are called basophilic rubricytes. As hemoglobin production continues and rough endoplasmic reticulum and ribosomes diminish, the cytoplasm becomes light blue or gray (polychromatophilic rubricytes) (*Figure 5*) or pink (normochromic rubricytes). Metarubricytes are the smallest nucleated erythroid cells. The nucleus has very condensed chromatin and the cytoplasm is gray or pink (*Figure 6*). The nucleus is extruded in the bone marrow. Further maturation occurs before the mature erythrocyte enters the blood by diapedesis through the endothelial cells that line the marrow sinusoids. A small amount of ineffective erythropoiesis occurs in normal animals. In ineffective erythropoiesis, developing erythroid cells in the bone marrow do not reach the final stages of maturation.

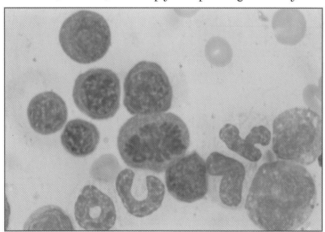

Figure 5. Erythroid precursors from the bone marrow of a dog with erythroid hyperplasia. Early erythroid precursors are characterized by round nuclei with condensed chromatin and intensely basophilic cytoplasm. Progressive condensation of the chromatin and formation of hemoglobin occur as the cells mature. Shown here are several stages of rubricyte development. There is one mitotic figure in the center and there are several myeloid precursors in the lower part of the field. Wright's stain, 1000X.

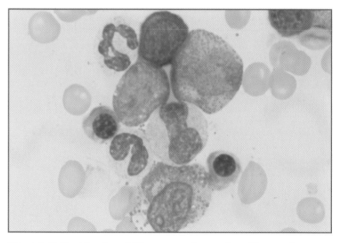

Figure 6. Erythroid and myeloid precursors from a dog with normal hematopoiesis. As hemoglobin concentration increases, the cytoplasm of erythroid precursors becomes light blue, then gray, and eventually a pink color that resembles the tintorial quality of mature erythrocytes. There are 2 partially hemaglobinized metarubricytes with gray cytoplasm and condensed nuclei on each side of this group of hematopoietic cells. A prorubricyte is present at the top. The remaining cells are myeloid precursors and a segmented neutrophil. Wright's stain, 1000X.

Megakaryocytopoiesis

Burst-forming units megakaryocyte (BFU-Meg) and CFU-Meg are the progenitor cells for megakaryocyte production. CFU-Meg divide and differentiate into megakaryoblasts, which are the earliest morphologically recognizable stage in the bone marrow. In contrast to cells of the myeloid and erythroid series, megakaryocytes increase in size with maturation. This occurs by endomitosis, in which the nucleus undergoes mitotic division but the cell itself does not divide. Megakaryoblasts initially are diploid cells with a single nucleus, but as the nucleus divides with cell maturation, they become polyploid cells with 2 or 4 nuclei. With progressive endomitosis and maturation, megakaryoblasts develop into promegakaryocytes and megakaryocytes. Nuclei of promegakaryocytes and megakaryocytes appear multilobed rather than as individual nuclei. The cytoplasm of mature megakaryocytes shows prominent azurophilic granulation. Mature megakaryocytes vary considerably in size, depending on the number of nuclear divisions that occurred prior to granule formation. Cytomorphologic features and sequence of maturation for megakaryocytic cells are listed in *Table 4*.

Megakaryoblasts are characterized by 1, 2, or 4 round nuclei with finely granular chromatin and 1 or more nucleoli (*Figure 7*). The nucleus occupies most of the cell. Megakaryoblast cytoplasm is deeply basophilic and nongranular. The cytoplasm may be vacuolated and some megakaryoblasts appear to have cytoplasmic blebs on the cell surface. These cells may be difficult to recognize mor-

phologically but can be identified by immunocytochemical staining for glycoprotein IIb-IIIa or platelet factor 4, or by cytochemical staining for acetylcholinesterase or platelet-specific peroxidase.

Promegakaryocytes have more than 4 nuclei and moderately basophilic agranular cytoplasm. Usually the nuclei are not clearly separated and appear instead as a multilobed structure (*Figure 8*). The cytoplasm is more abundant than in megakaryoblasts so the nuclear to cytoplasmic ratio is lower. As maturation continues, the nucleus becomes more lobulated and the chromatin becomes more condensed. Focal areas of fine, azurophilic granules develop in the

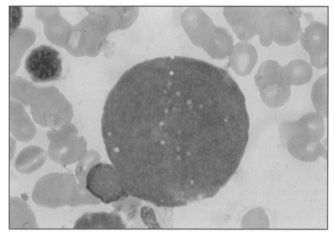

Figure 7. Megakaryoblast from a dog with megakaryocytic hyperplasia. Megakaryoblasts are larger than myeloblasts and rubriblasts and are characterized by 1, 2, or 4 nuclei (as in this cell) with finely granular chromatin and nucleoli. The cytoplasm is very basophilic at this early stage of development. Wright's stain, 1000X.

Table 4. Cytomorphologic Features and Sequence of Maturation of Megakaryocytic Cells in the Bone Marrow

Cell	Cytomorphologic Features	Cell	Cytomorphologic Features
Megakaryoblast *Figure 7*	• Larger than myeloblast or rubriblast • 1 to 4 distinct nuclei • Small amount of deeply basophilic cytoplasm • Cytoplasmic blebs may be present on the cell periphery	Megakaryocyte *Figure 9*	• Cell size varies with number of nuclear divisions • Abundant, pale blue cytoplasm with numerous small, pinkish-purple granules
Promegakaryocyte *Figure 8*	• 8 or more nuclei • Nuclei often appear fused together • Small amount of deeply to moderately basophilic cytoplasm	Platelets	• Vary in size and shape • Non-nucleated cytoplasmic fragments of megakaryocytes • Light blue cytoplasm with numerous small, pinkish-purple granules

Modified from: Raskin RE. Myelopoiesis and myeloproliferative disorders. *Vet Clin North Am Small Anim Prac.* September, 1996;1030.

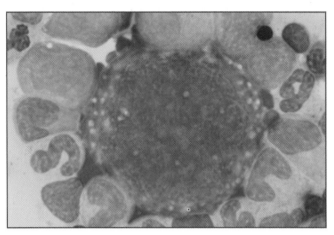

Figure 8. Promegakaryocyte from a dog with megakaryocytic hyperplasia. The nuclei appear as a homogeneous mass. The cytoplasm is still very basophilic. The cytoplasmic vacuoles and blebs on the periphery sometimes are seen in megakaryocytic cells. Wright's stain, 1000X.

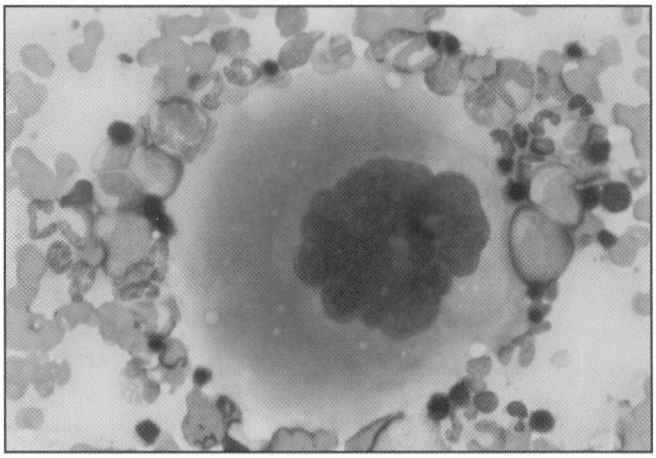

Figure 9. Mature megakaryocyte from a dog with megakaryocytic hyperplasia. Mature megakaryocytes are very large and are easily seen with the low power objective. Abundant granular cytoplasm and multilobed nuclei are characteristic features of mature megakaryocytes. Wright's stain, 400X.

cytoplasm and the cytoplasm becomes less basophilic.

Megakaryocytes are the largest hematopoietic cells in the bone marrow (20-160 microns in diameter) and are characterized by a single, multilobed nuclear mass, and abundant, pale-staining cytoplasm with numerous, small, azurophilic granules (*Figure 9*). Pseudopod-like projections of cytoplasm called proplatelets penetrate through sinusoidal endothelial cells and into the marrow sinusoids, where they break away from the megakaryocyte to form platelets. Platelets also may be formed by fragmentation of megakaryocyte cytoplasm and surface blebbing or budding.

Megakaryocytopoiesis is regulated by platelet mass. Thrombocytopenia leads to increases in megakaryocyte number, mitotic indices, nuclear ploidy, and cell size, and a decrease in megakaryocyte maturation time. Megakaryocytopoiesis and thrombopoiesis are stimulated by thrombopoietin, IL-3, GM-CSF, and IL-6. IL-6 increases in inflammation and may explain the thrombocytosis

seen in patients with ongoing inflammation.

Lymphopoiesis

Pluripotential lymphoid progenitors give rise to B-cell progenitors and T-cell progenitors. B and T lymphocytes appear similar morphologically but can be identified by different distribution in lymphoid tissues, surface receptors and antigens, and functional characteristics. B-cell progenitors produce B-cells in the bone marrow in most mammals. B cells then migrate to lymph nodes, spleen, and mucosal surfaces. Most T cell differentiation occurs outside the bone marrow. T-cell progenitors exit the bone marrow and migrate to the thymus. After maturation in the thymus, T cells migrate to lymph nodes, spleen, and mucosal surfaces. Natural killer (NK) cells likely develop from T-cell progenitors and undergo maturation in the bone marrow and thymus.

Chapter 2: Indications for Bone Marrow Evaluation

Evaluation of the bone marrow is indicated when hematologic abnormalities are observed in the peripheral blood, and there is inadequate information provided by the CBC and other tests to make a diagnosis. Common indications for bone marrow aspiration are persistent and unexplained non-regenerative anemia, neutropenia, or thrombocytopenia. In general, it is inappropriate to perform a marrow aspirate on dogs and cats with regenerative anemias. In non-regenerative anemia, it is important that extra-marrow causes of suppression, such as chronic inflammatory disease, iron deficiency, chronic renal disease, or endocrinopathies (eg, hypothyroidism), be ruled out prior to subjecting the patient to a bone marrow aspirate or biopsy.

Bicytopenias, pancytopenias, or abnormal circulating cells usually warrant examination of the bone marrow. Unexplained increases of immature blood cells in the circulation may require a marrow aspirate in order to evaluate dysplasias in these cell lines. Examples include increased numbers of nucleated erythrocytes without polychromasia and reticulocytosis, a neutrophilic left shift without an apparent cause of inflammation, or persistent thrombocytosis with large or dysplastic-appearing platelets. Inappropriate increases in nucleated red blood cells (nRBC) with a neutrophilic left shift are called a leukoerythroblastic reaction. Bone marrow examination may be

Common Indications for Bone Marrow Aspiration

- ❏ Non-regenerative anemia
- ❏ Neutropenia
- ❏ Thrombocytopenia
- ❏ Abnormal circulating cells

used to evaluate a patient for a suspected hematopoietic neoplasm, such as myeloid or lymphoid leukemia, plasma cell neoplasms, or malignant histiocytosis. It may also be helpful in staging tumors, such as lymphoma and mast cell tumors.

Other indications for performance of a bone marrow aspirate include evaluation of patients with hyperproteinemia and/or hypercalcemia for diseases such as multiple myeloma, lymphoma, or other neoplasms that have metastasized to the bone. Bone marrow aspirates may also prove fruitful in identifying infectious agents such as *Histoplasma capsulatum, Leishmania infantum,* or *Cytauxzoon felis.*

Chapter 3: Procedures for Bone Marrow Aspiration and Biopsy

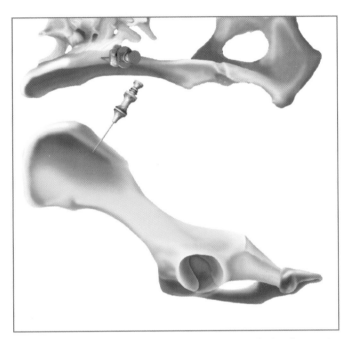

Figure 1. Dorsal (top) and lateral (bottom) views of the site for placement of the needle to obtain bone marrow from the iliac crest. This site may be used for medium to large dogs. (Illustration by Tim Vojt.)

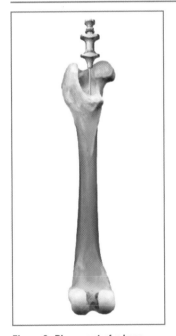

Figure 2. Placement of a bone marrow needle in the trochanteric fossa of the femur. This site may be used in cats and smaller dogs. (Illustration by Tim Vojt.)

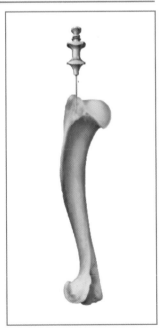

Figure 3. This site for obtaining bone marrow from the humerus also may be used in small dogs and cats. (Illustration by Tim Vojt.)

Bone Marrow Aspiration Technique

The iliac crest is the primary site for collection of bone marrow in medium and large dogs (*Figure 1*). In cats and small dogs, the trochanteric fossa of the femur (*Figure 2*) or proximal humerus (*Figure 3*) may be used. Direct aspiration of lytic bone lesions may also be performed.

Bone marrow aspiration should be performed as a sterile procedure. The area should be clipped and surgically prepared. All instruments and needles should be sterilized. It is often not necessary to use general anesthesia. Bone marrow frequently can be collected after a local anesthetic is injected in the overlying skin and periosteum; however, some patients may require sedation, in addition to manual restraint.

Once the area is prepared and the local anesthetic is administered, a small stab incision with a scalpel blade is made through the skin over the site. A bone marrow aspirate needle should be 16- to 18-gauge and 1 to 1-3/4 inches in length. It should have a stylet that can be locked in place during advancement through the cortical bone (*Figure 4*), which prevents plugging of the needle. Needles that are commonly used include Rosenthal and Illinois reusable needles and Monoject™ (Sherwood Medical, St. Louis, MO) disposable needles. Once in place, the needle is slowly rotated under pressure until it is through the cortex and firmly seated in the bone. The stylet can then be removed. Using a 12 to 20 cc syringe, apply only enough suction to aspirate 1 to 2 drops of marrow into the syringe. Aspiration of larger quantities of marrow usually results in hemodilution of the sample.

Because bone marrow clots rapidly, mixing with an anticoagulant (eg, EDTA) is recommended. The sample should be placed into a small purple top vacutainer tube from which the excess EDTA has been shaken out. Alternatively, several drops

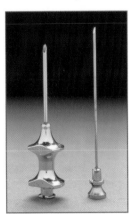

Figure 4. A Rosenthal needle for bone marrow aspirates with a stylet that may be locked in place.

of EDTA may be drawn into the syringe prior to sampling. If the sample is not mixed with an anticoagulant, smears for cytology should be made immediately. Marrow smears can be made as pull or push preparations (*Figures 5 and 6*). If the sample is hemodiluted, it may be possible to isolate the particles of marrow by placing the sample on a slide or in a small petri dish and tilting the sample to allow excess blood to run off. The spicules may then be picked up on a clean slide and smeared. Air-dried smears may be sent to a reference lab for additional processing or may be stained in house with Wright's stain or a commercial quick stain for microscopic evaluation.

Bone Marrow Core Biopsy Technique

Core biopsies of bone marrow may also be obtained for histopathologic evaluation. The most common site for obtaining a core biopsy is the iliac crest; however, biopsies also may be taken of specific lesions. Like the aspiration technique, the biopsy procedure should be performed under sterile conditions and may be done using local anesthesia. A larger Jamshidi bone marrow biopsy needle (11- to 14-gauge) with lockable stylet is pushed through the cortical bone as described earlier. The stylet is removed and the needle advanced several millimeters into the trabecular bone. The needle should then be slightly retracted and advanced several times to loosen the core from the boney cortex. The needle is then backed out of the bone. The core is pushed from the needle using the stylet and may be used to make impression or rolled smears for cytology, or placed in formalin for histologic processing. It is important to make the smears for cytology away from the formalin container because formalin fumes can interfere with stain-

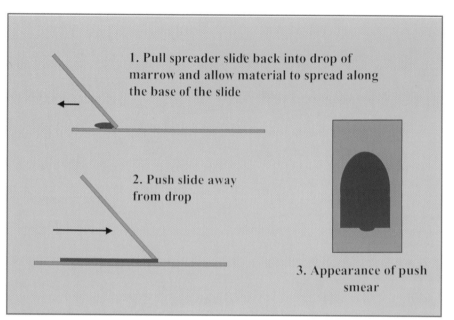

1. Pull spreader slide back into drop of marrow and allow material to spread along the base of the slide

2. Push slide away from drop

3. Appearance of push smear

Figure 5. The technique for making a push smear. This method is commonly used for preparing blood films.

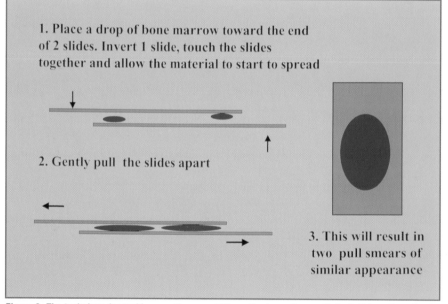

1. Place a drop of bone marrow toward the end of 2 slides. Invert 1 slide, touch the slides together and allow the material to start to spread

2. Gently pull the slides apart

3. This will result in two pull smears of similar appearance

Figure 6. The technique for making a pull smear. This method usually results in 2 slides of good quality and may result in less breakage of cells during preparation.

ing of the cytologic specimen. Once the bone in the sample is decalcified, core biopsies may be embedded and stained. Embedding of the fixed bone marrow specimen in paraffin often results in shrinkage artifact that may distort the cells. Use of plastic embedding will reduce this problem; however, plastic embedding is not as widely available as paraffin embedding.

Chapter 4: Cytologic and Histologic Evaluation of the Bone Marrow

Cytologic Evaluation of the Bone Marrow

Cytologic evaluation of the bone marrow involves scanning the smear with a low power (10×) objective and making detailed observations with a high power (100×, oil immersion) objective. The 10× objective is used to estimate cellularity, to evaluate megakaryocyte number and maturation, and to locate an area to examine with higher magnification. The 100× objective is used to evaluate cytomorphologic features, to determine the myeloid to erythroid ratio (M:E ratio), to evaluate synchrony and completeness of maturation of the myeloid and erythroid lineages, to determine the numbers of lymphocytes and plasma cells, and to assess iron status. Other normal cells, abnormal cells, and etiologic agents also are identified under high power.

It is critical to use the 10× objective to locate appropriate areas for 100× evaluation by finding highly cellular places on the slide where the cells are intact and occur in a single layer (*Figure 1*). Evaluation of areas that are too thick or in which the cells are broken will result in misinterpretation. Appropriate areas may occur around spicules, along the sides of the smear, or near the feathered edge. Several areas usually are selected for detailed observation using the 100× objective.

Estimation of cellularity is difficult unless bone spicules are present. Spicules (or particles) appear as dark, blue-staining areas when the slide is viewed grossly (*Figure 2*). When examined microscopically, they contain hematopoietic precursors, adipocytes, and small blood vessels. If bone spicules are present, the relative amount of hematopoietic cells and adipocytes is determined. Normally, 30% to 50% of the spicule is occupied by hematopoietic cells and 50% to 70% of the spicule is occupied by adipocytes.

Cellularity appears increased if hematopoietic cells are greater than 50% of the particle, indicating that the bone marrow is hyperplastic (*Figure 3*). Myelophthisis is the term used when cellularity appears increased from macrophages or neoplastic cells that have replaced normal hematopoietic cells. Cellularity appears decreased if adipocytes are greater than 70% of the spicule, and this occurs when the bone marrow is hypoplastic or aplastic (*Figure 4*). When there is concern that bone marrow hypoplasia or aplasia is present, cellularity is best evaluated on histologic section.

The number of megakaryocytes is affected by the amount of hemodilution. Usually, at least 2 to 10 megakaryocytes are present per smear. Megakaryocytes often are associated with bone marrow spicules. Typically, 2 to 7 megakaryocytes are present per spicule (*Figure 5*). Megakaryocytic hyperplasia is reflected as increased numbers of megakaryocytes. Megakaryocyte numbers may

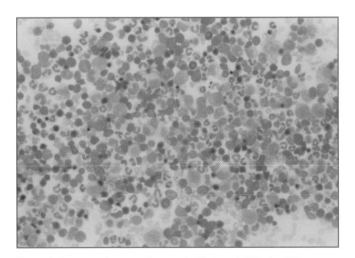

Figure 1. An appropriate counting area is illustrated. This should be a cellular area in which the cells are intact and occur as a single layer of cells. Thicker areas and areas in which the cells are broken should be avoided. Wright's stain, 200X.

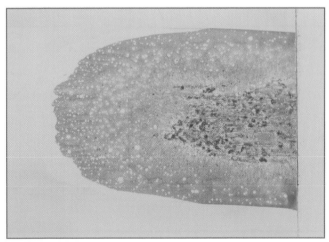

Figure 2. Bone marrow smear from a dog illustrating numerous blue-staining areas at the base of the smear. These represent spicules or particles of bone and are an indication that an adequate sample was collected. Wright's stain.

appear decreased if there is hemodilution or decreased production.

Immature megakaryocytic cells (megakaryoblasts) are large cells with 1 to 4 distinct nuclei, deeply basophilic cytoplasm, and no cytoplasmic granules (*Figure 6*). Small cytoplasmic blebs may be present around the periphery of the cytoplasm. As megakaryocytes mature, the nucleus continues to divide but the cytoplasm does not, in a process called endomitosis. Mature megakaryocytes are very large cells with multiple nuclei that most often appear fused. They have abundant granular cytoplasm (*Figure 7*).

The myeloid to erythroid (M:E) ratio is a numerical esti-

mate of the relative numbers of myeloid (granulocyte and monocyte) precursors and erythroid (red blood cell) precursors. The terms "myeloid" and "granulocytic" are sometimes used interchangeably because granulocytes are much more numerous than monocytes and changes in the myeloid fraction are most often due to changes in the number of granulocytes. Granulocytes include precursors of neutrophils, eosinophils, and basophils. The M:E ratio can be determined by dividing the total number of granulocytic cells by the total number of nucleated erythroid cells obtained on a differential count of 500 nucleated bone mar-

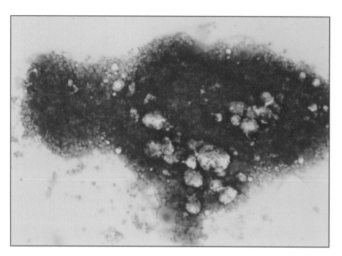

Figure 3. Hypercellular spicule from a dog with acute myeloid leukemia. Greater than 50% of the spicule is occupied by hematopoietic cells and less than 50% of the spicule is occupied by adipocytes. Wright's stain, 100X.

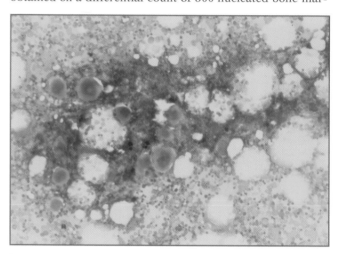

Figure 5. Megakaryocytes associated with a spicule of bone marrow from a dog with mild megakaryocytic hyperplasia. Typically, 2 to 7 megakaryocytes are present per spicule. There are 9 megakaryocytes associated with this spicule. Megakaryocyte number is easily evaluated with low power magnification because the cells are very large. Wright's stain, 100X.

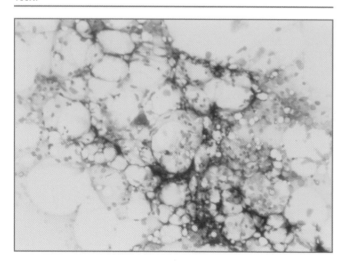

Figure 4. Hypocellular particle from a dog with pancytopenia of undetermined etiology. Less than 30% of the spicule is occupied by hematopoietic cells and more than 70% of the spicule is occupied by adipocytes. Wright's stain, 100X.

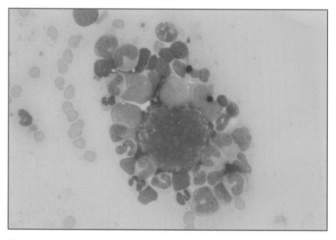

Figure 6. Immature megakaryocyte surrounded by myeloid and erythroid precursors. Notice how much larger the megakaryocytic cell is than the other hematopoietic precursors. The minimal amount of basophilic, agranular cytoplasm is characteristic of immature megakaryocytes. Wright's stain, 400X.

row cells. Megakaryocytes, lymphocytes, plasma cells, macrophages, mast cells, endothelial cells, adipocytes, osteoclasts, and osteoblasts are excluded from the calculation of the M:E ratio. Bone marrow differential cell counts are very time consuming. As an alternative to a differential cell count, a satisfactory estimate of the M:E ratio often can be obtained by simply classifying cells as myeloid or erythroid, rather than identifying each cell as a particular stage of differentiation.

Nuclear and cytoplasmic characteristics, rather than cell size, are used to classify myeloid and erythroid cells. Myeloid cells are characterized by round, oval, indented or segmented nuclei; finely stippled chromatin; and lightly basophilic cytoplasm with primary or secondary granules (*Figure 8*). Erythroid cells are characterized by round nuclei with condensed chromatin and intensely basophilic cytoplasm with no cytoplasmic granules (*Figure 9*).

The normal M:E ratio varies with species and is 0.75 to 2.5 (mean = 1.3) in dogs and 1.0 to 3.0 (mean = 1.6) in cats. The correct interpretation of the M:E ratio depends on the evaluation of a concurrent CBC. A normal M:E ratio could mean that myelopoiesis and erythropoiesis are normal or that there is both granulocytic and erythroid hyperplasia or hypoplasia (*Figure 10*). Changes in the M:E ratio may be helpful in establishing a differential diagnosis.

An increased M:E ratio with no maturation abnormalities can occur with granulocytic hyperplasia, erythroid hypoplasia, or both. An increased M:E ratio with few

mature granulocytic cells present in the bone marrow aspirate may indicate that there is marked inflammation and the mature granulocytes are exiting the marrow very quickly. This is sometimes referred to as depletion of the granulocyte reserve. Alternatively, a hypercellular marrow with predominantly immature granulocytes may indicate that there is a maturation arrest, and granulocytic leukemia would be a differential diagnosis. In either case, erythroid hypoplasia often is present concurrently.

A decreased M:E ratio usually indicates increased erythrocyte production in response to a shortened red blood

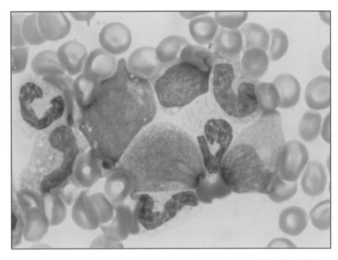

Figure 8. Myeloid cells from a dog with normal hematopoiesis. Myeloid cells are characterized by round, oval, indented, or segmented nuclei; finely stippled chromatin; and lightly basophilic cytoplasm with primary or secondary granules. Wright's stain, 1000X.

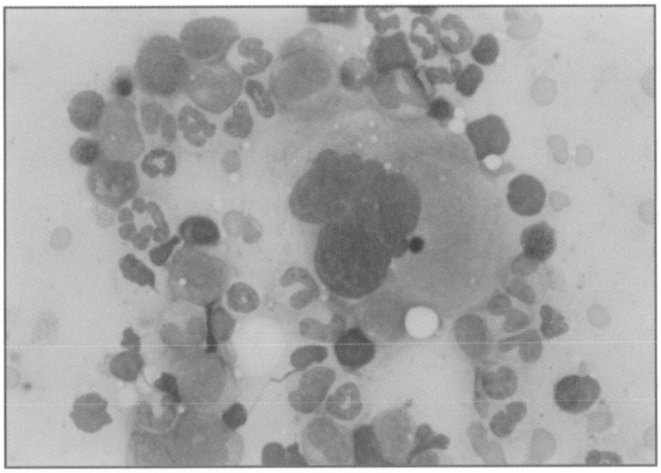

Figure 7. Mature megakaryocyte surrounded by myeloid and erythroid precursors. Notice the abundant granular cytoplasm compared to the immature megakaryocyte in the previous figure. Wright's stain, 400X.

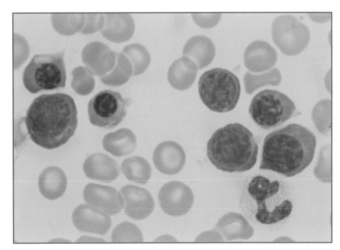

Figure 9. Erythroid cells from a dog with normal hematopoiesis. Erythroid cells are characterized by round nuclei, condensed chromatin, and basophilic, agranular cytoplasm. Wright's stain, 1000X.

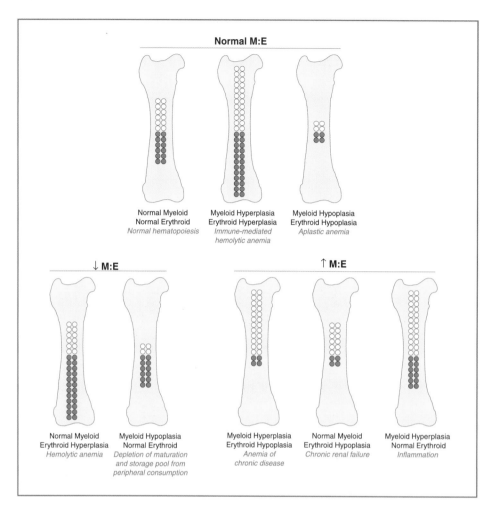

Normal M:E

Normal Myeloid
Normal Erythroid
Normal hematopoiesis

Myeloid Hyperplasia
Erythroid Hyperplasia
*Immune-mediated
hemolytic anemia*

Myeloid Hypoplasia
Erythroid Hypoplasia
Aplastic anemia

↓ M:E

Normal Myeloid
Erythroid Hyperplasia
Hemolytic anemia

Myeloid Hypoplasia
Normal Erythroid
*Depletion of maturation
and storage pool from
peripheral consumption*

↑ M:E

Myeloid Hyperplasia
Erythroid Hypoplasia
*Anemia of
chronic disease*

Normal Myeloid
Erythroid Hypoplasia
Chronic renal failure

Myeloid Hyperplasia
Normal Erythroid
Inflammation

Figure 10. Schematic of myeloid to erythroid (M:E) ratios. Myeloid cells are indicated by the white circles and erythroid cells are indicated by the red circles. The normal M:E ratio is 0.75 to 2.5 in dogs and 1.0 to 3.0 in cats. The illustration depicts normal, decreased, and increased M:E ratios, and mechanisms associated with each kind of change. Examples of diseases that might be associated with each type of mechanism are indicated in red. (Illustration by Tim Vojt.)

cell (RBC) lifespan, as in hemolytic anemia. A decreased M:E rarely indicates selective depression of granulocytes, but may result from rapid depletion of the granulocyte storage and maturation pools when peripheral consumption of granulocytes is greatly increased. This may be difficult to document with only one CBC.

The myeloid (granulocytic) and erythroid cell lines should be evaluated for an orderly sequence of maturation. Myeloblasts and rubriblasts are the earliest recognizable precursor cells of the myeloid and erythroid lineages, respectively. Less than 2% of all nucleated cells (ANC) in the bone marrow should be myeloblasts and rubriblasts. These cells divide and differentiate as shown in *Figure 11*, forming a "pyramid" with few blast cells at the apex and numerous differentiated cells at the base. This is referred to

as "orderly maturation."

The most mature nucleated cells in the bone marrow (segmented/band neutrophils for myeloid cells; metarubricytes for erythroid cells) should be present in the highest numbers. This is referred to as "completeness of maturation." Small numbers of a more mature cell stage relative to a less mature stage is referred to as a "maturation arrest," and may reflect increased consumption of more mature elements or a defect in cell maturation.

Increased numbers of immature hematopoietic cells may occur with erythroid, myeloid, or megakaryocytic hyperplasia, in which case blast cells usually are still less than 2% of ANC. Immature hematopoietic cells also may be increased in dysplastic or neoplastic disorders, such as lymphoma or leukemia. Hematopoietic blast cells in dysplastic or neoplastic disorders exceed 2% of ANC. The diagnosis of these disorders is discussed in Chapters 5 and 6. Morphologic abnormalities in any of the cells should be noted. These may include cytoplasmic vacuolation, asynchrony of nuclear and cytoplasmic maturation (megaloblastic cells), binucleate cells, giant nuclear forms, and abnormal nuclear shapes.

Lymphocytes usually are less than 10% and 15% of ANC in bone marrow aspirates from healthy dogs and cats, respectively. Lymphocytes in the bone marrow resemble small lymphocytes in the peripheral blood and are characterized by a round nucleus with moderately clumped chromatin and a narrow rim of pale cytoplasm (*Figure 12*). Nucleoli usually are not apparent. It may be difficult to distinguish small lymphocytes from metarubricytes. Lymphocytes usually have a higher nuclear to cytoplasmic ratio, less condensed chromatin, and lighter staining cytoplasm. Lymphocytes increase in number when there is lymphoid

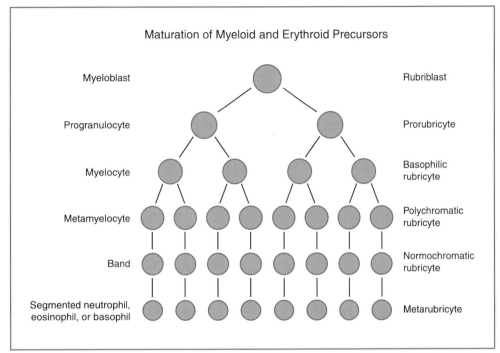

Maturation of Myeloid and Erythroid Precursors

Myeloblast — Rubriblast

Progranulocyte — Prorubricyte

Myelocyte — Basophilic rubricyte

Metamyelocyte — Polychromatic rubricyte

Band — Normochromatic rubricyte

Segmented neutrophil, eosinophil, or basophil — Metarubricyte

Figure 11. Schematic representation of maturation of myeloid and erythroid precursors showing the "pyramid" effect of very few immature precursors forming the apex of the pyramid and numerous differentiated cells forming the base of the pyramid. This is an indication of orderly maturation that progresses to completion. (Illustration by Tim Vojt.)

usually are less than 2% of ANC. Plasma cells usually are round or oval and have abundant basophilic cytoplasm and an eccentrically located round nucleus. The nuclear chromatin appears very condensed with interspersed light areas. There often is a perinuclear pale area in the cytoplasm that represents the Golgi apparatus (*Figure 13*). Occasionally, the cytoplasm is filled with round or angular structures called Russell bodies (*Figure 14*). These structures usually are clear or pale and likely are distended rough endoplasmic reticulum. Plasma cells with abundant Russell bodies are called Mott cells. Plasma cells increase in number when

hyperplasia or lymphoid neoplasia.

Occasional plasma cells may be present in bone marrow aspirates from healthy dogs and cats. In the absence of antigenic stimulation or plasma cell neoplasia, plasma cells

there is antigenic stimulation or plasma cell neoplasia (multiple myeloma). It may be difficult to distinguish plasma cells from polychromatophilic rubricytes. Plasma cells usually are larger, have a smaller nuclear to cytoplasmic ratio,

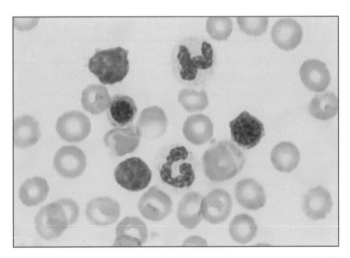

Figure 12. Bone marrow from a dog with normal hematopoiesis showing 2 segmented neutrophils, 1 metarubricyte, 1 rubricyte, and 2 small lymphocytes. Lymphocytes have a higher nuclear to cytoplasmic ratio, less condensed chromatin, and lighter staining cytoplasm than metarubricytes. The lymphocyte in the upper left is broken but a narrow rim of cytoplasm can be seen on the left side of the lymphocyte on the lower left. A metarubricyte is located between these 2 lymphocytes. Wright's stain, 1000X.

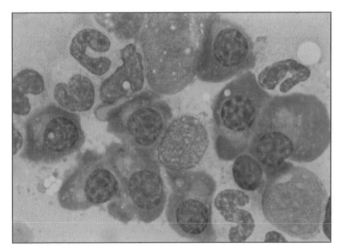

Figure 13. Plasma cells from the bone marrow of a dog with plasma cell hyperplasia. Plasma cells are large, round to oval cells with abundant basophilic cytoplasm and an eccentrically placed nucleus. There often is a perinuclear clear zone, which is very prominent in the plasma cells shown here. This likely represents the Golgi area. Wright's stain, 1000X.

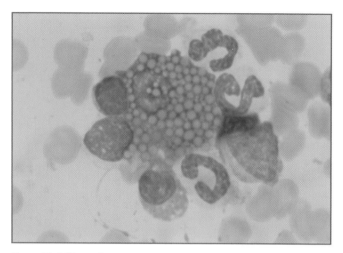

Figure 14. A Mott cell from the bone marrow of a dog with plasma cell hyperplasia. The round, pale structures are called Russell bodies and likely represent rough endoplasmic reticulum distended with antibody. Wright's stain, 1000X.

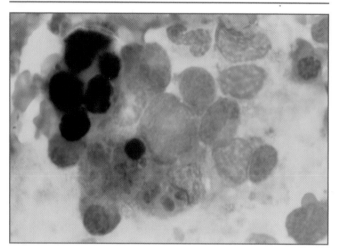

Figure 15. Two macrophages distended with hemosiderin are shown in this figure. Occasional macrophages are present in bone marrow smears from healthy animals, but they may be difficult to recognize unless they have phagocytized cells or etiologic agents or contain pigment granules, as shown here. Wright's stain, 1000X.

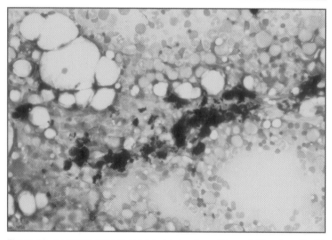

Figure 16. A spicule of bone marrow from a dog with myeloid and erythroid hyperplasia. The clear spaces associated with the spicule represent the cytoplasm of adipocytes. The nucleus often is difficult to visualize. Wright's stain, 100X.

an eccentrically placed nucleus, and have a more bluish hue to the cytoplasm.

Other cells, which may be present in small numbers in normal marrow, include macrophages, adipocytes, osteoclasts, osteoblasts, endothelial cells, and mast cells. Macrophages are less than 2% of ANC in bone marrow from healthy dogs and cats. They usually are characterized by abundant cytoplasm and a round to irregularly shaped nucleus. Macrophages may be difficult to recognize unless they have phagocytized pyknotic nuclei, cells, or etiologic agents, or contain hemosiderin (*Figure 15*). Macrophages may increase in number if there is immune-mediated hemolytic anemia, granulomatous inflammation, bone marrow necrosis, or hemophagocytic syndrome. A neoplastic proliferation of macrophages occurs in animals with malignant histiocytosis.

Adipocytes occur in bone marrow aspirates but often are difficult to identify because the fixation and staining process disrupts the cell membrane and dissolves the lipid content. Intact adipocytes may be recognized in small spicules of trabecular bone, which frequently occur in bone marrow aspirates (*Figure 16*). Adipocytes are characterized by abundant, clear cytoplasm and small, round, eccentrically placed nuclei. Spicule-associated adipocytes may appear decreased in erythroid and myeloid hyperplasia and may appear increased in hypoplastic or aplastic disorders.

Only rare osteoclasts and osteoblasts are present in normal bone marrow aspirate smears. Osteoclasts are large, irregularly-shaped cells with abundant pinkish granular cytoplasm. Osteoclasts are similar in size to megakaryocytes, but osteoclasts have multiple oval nuclei that appear to be separated within the cytoplasm, in contrast to the multiple, fused nuclei in megakaryocytes (*Figure 17*). Osteoblasts are characterized by a round to oval shape, abundant cytoplasm, and a round to oval eccentrically located nucleus.

Endothelial cells may be present in some bone marrow aspirates. They are characterized by their elongated shape, narrow nucleus, and abundant pale eosinophilic cytoplasm (*Figure 18*). Often small aggregates of endothelial cells are present, which likely represent fragments of the bone marrow vascular sinuses.

Occasional mast cells may be present in bone marrow from healthy dogs and cats. Mast cells are large, round cells with round nuclei and abundant cytoplasm. The characteristic morphologic feature of mast cells is the presence of numerous metachromatic (purple) granules dispersed throughout the cytoplasm (*Figure 19*). Mast cells usually are less than 1 per 1000 nucleated cells. Increased numbers of mast cells can occur with some inflammatory diseases, in aplastic anemia, and in neoplastic proliferations of mast cells.

Iron is stored as hemosiderin in the bone marrow and appears as dark green to black amorphous granules with Wright's stain (*Figure 20*). Hemosiderin usually is associated with spicules and may appear intracellular or extracellular. Hemosiderin often can be visualized in bone marrow aspirates from healthy dogs but rarely is present in bone marrow from cats. The presence of hemosiderin indicates adequate iron stores. Prussian blue staining can be used to increase the sensitivity of detecting stainable iron. In dogs with iron deficiency anemia, stainable iron is undetectable. It is difficult to evaluate stainable iron in cats because hemosiderin is not usually detectable; however, iron deficiency in cats is very uncommon. Other more sensitive assays are available to evaluate iron status in dogs and cats. Hemosiderin may appear increased in dogs with hemolytic anemia or anemia associated with inflammatory disease, due to increased erythrophagocytosis or abnormal accumulation in macrophages, respectively.

Histologic Evaluation of Bone Marrow

For routine bone marrow assessment, aspiration and cytology are the preferred method and are best for evalua-

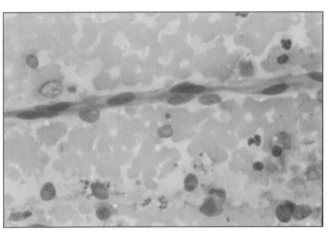

Figure 18. An aggregate of endothelial cells from part of a small blood vessel. Endothelial cells are characterized by their elongated shape and narrow nucleus. Wright's stain, 400X.

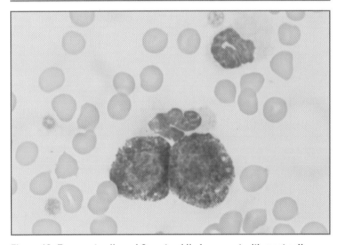

Figure 19. Two mast cells and 2 neutrophils from a cat with mast cell leukemia. Mast cells are recognized by their prominent cytoplasmic granules, which stain purple with Wright's stain. The round nucleus may be obscured if the granules are numerous. 1000X.

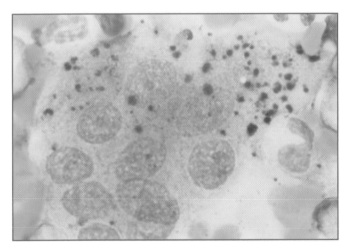

Figure 17. An osteoclast from a dog with normal hematopoiesis. Osteoclasts are recognized infrequently. Like megakaryocytes, they are very large cells with abundant cytoplasm, but osteoclasts have multiple nuclei that appear separated from each other, in contrast to the multilobed nuclei in megakaryocytes. The cytoplasmic granules present in this cell sometimes are seen in osteoclasts and these are much larger than the granules in megakaryocytes. Wright's stain, 1000X.

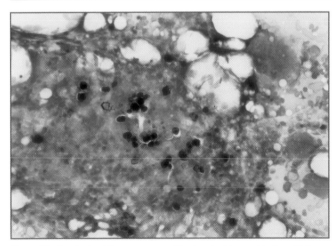

Figure 20. A spicule of bone marrow with abundant hemosiderin, which appears as dark greenish black granules. Hemosiderin is an iron-protein complex that is stored in macrophages as a source of iron for erythropoiesis. Wright's stain, 100X.

tion of hematopoietic precursors. However, there are circumstances in which histologic evaluation of core biopsies can provide useful information, such as evaluating cellularity of the marrow, assessing architectural changes such as myelofibrosis, determining the cause of repeatedly unsuccessful marrow aspirates, staging of neoplastic processes, or detecting the presence and extent of infiltrative disease. Core biopsies can also be taken of specific lytic lesions to help determine pathogenesis. Histologic sections of bone marrow can be used for special staining techniques such as iron staining for evaluation of iron stores or for immunophenotyping of hematopoietic tumors.

Assessment of cellularity of a core biopsy is expressed as a percentage (*Figure 21*). Normal bone marrow should contain 30% to 50% hematopoietic precursors and 50% to 70% fat, depending on age of the patient and site from which the sample was taken. Very young animals may have up to 100% cellularity. Bone marrow adipocytes, fibroblasts, macrophages and vascular sinuses form a supporting network for the blood forming elements. The bone marrow does not contain lymphatics.

The blood forming elements are found as clusters of cells interspersed among the fat and trabecular bone (*Figure 22*). Erythroid and megakaryocytic progenitors are found along the vascular sinuses, whereas granulocytic precursors are formed in clusters, distant to the sinuses. As granulocytes mature, they become mobile and are able to migrate from their site of production to the vascular sinus in order

to attain access to the circulation. Production of lymphocytes takes place along the endosteum of the bone lamellae. In cases of inflammation and antigenic stimulation, clusters of lymphocytes and plasma cells may be observed.

Cytochemical Stains

Although routine Romanowsky staining allows correct identification of most normal and abnormal cells in the bone marrow, special cytochemical and immunocytochemical stains sometimes are used to identify atypical or poorly differentiated cells, especially in animals with leukemia (*Table 1*). Cytochemical stains may be helpful in identifying granulocytic and monocytic cells but are not very useful in identifying lymphoid cells or erythroid precursors, because the latter 2 lineages most often exhibit negative staining patterns.

Immunophenotyping

Immunophenotyping has enhanced accurate cell identification for classification of hematopoietic cells. Many monoclonal antibodies have been developed that bind to "cluster of differentiation" (CD) antigens, which occur on the surface of many hematopoietic cells. Numerous CD antigens have been characterized and the pattern of distribution on the cell surface often helps determine cell lineage and stage of differentiation. Leukocyte immunophenotyping has been very helpful in the classification of hematopoietic neoplasms in human beings and may have similar applications in veterinary medicine. Common markers for leukocytes are listed

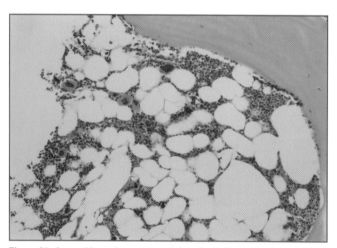

Figure 21. A core biopsy from a normal dog illustrating approximately 50% cellularity. H&E stain, 100X.

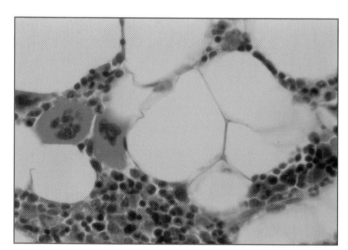

Figure 22. A core biopsy from a normal dog showing hematopoietic elements interspersed with fat. Two mature megakaryocytes are seen and are the largest of the blood forming elements. Iron stores may be seen as brown pigment. H&E stain, 400X.

in *Table 2*. In many cases, antibodies developed against human antigens cross-react with dog and cat hematopoietic cells. However, some antibodies are species-specific and the distribution of antigens on specific cell types may differ. Lineage infidelity and expression of antigens normally not present have been reported in neoplastic cells.

Table 1. Cytochemical and Immunocytochemical Staining Reactions for Leukemias in Dogs and Cats

Stain	Myelogenous	Myelomonocytic	Monocytic	Lymphocytic	Erythroid	Megakaryocytic
ACE	-	-	-	-	-	+
ALP	+	+	-	+[1]	-	-
ANBE	-	+	+[2]	+[3]	-	+/-
ANBE with fluoride	-	-	-	+[3]	-	+/-
BG	-	-	+[4]	+[4]	-	-
CAE	+	+	-	-	-	+/-
FVIIIRAg	-	-	-	-	-	+
OMX	+[5]	-	-	-	-	-
PO	+	+	-	-	-	+[6]
SBB	+	+	-	-	-	-

ACE	Acetylcholinesterase	FVIIIRAg	Factor VIII-related antigen (von Willebrand's)
ALP	Alkaline phosphatase	OMX	Omegaexonuclease
ANBE	Alpha naphthyl butyrate esterase (or nonspecific esterase)	PO	Peroxidase
BG	Beta-glucuronidase	SBB	Sudan black B
CAE	Chloracetate esterase (or specific esterase)		

[1] Present in some cases of canine B-cell lymphoma and feline lymphoma involving large granular lymphocytes

[2] Diffuse staining pattern

[3] Occasionally positive with a focal or granular pattern; reaction not inhibited by fluoride

[4] Monocytes have a finely granular pattern; T lymphocytes have a focal pattern

[5] Specific for basophilic differentiation

[6] Positive for platelet peroxidase at the ultrastructural level

Modified from: Raskin RE. Myelopoiesis and myeloproliferative disorders. *Vet Clin North Am Small Anim Prac.* September, 1996;1047.

Table 2. Selected Cluster Differentiation (CD) Antigens for Dog and Cat Leukocytes

CD Antigen	Cell Population Identified
CD3	Mature T lymphocytes
CD4	Helper T lymphocytes; granulocytes (dogs)
CD8	Suppressor T lymphocytes
CD14	Monocytes
CD19, CD20	Total B lymphocytes
CD21	Mature B lymphocytes
CD16, CD56, CD57	Natural killer (NK) cells, cytotoxic T lymphocytes
CD34	Hematopoietic stem cells

Part II

Chapter 5: **Evaluation of Abnormal Bone Marrow**

Hyperplasia

- ❑ Erythroid hyperplasia

- ❑ Granulocytic hyperplasia

- ❑ Monocyte/macrophage hyperplasia

- ❑ Megakaryocytic hyperplasia

- ❑ Lymphocytic/plasma cell hyperplasia

Erythroid Hyperplasia

Enhanced production of erythroid precursors is the normal response in diseases in which there is either increased loss of erythrocytes through hemorrhage or increased destruction of erythrocytes (shortened red cell life span or hemolysis). Erythroid hyperplasia also occurs in cases of polycythemia and is discussed in chapter 6. Both hemorrhagic and hemolytic processes should be accompanied by increased release of reticulocytes into the peripheral blood. Absolute reticulocyte counts of greater than 60,000/µl in dogs and greater than 50,000/µl in cats suggest a regenerative response. The increase in reticulocyte count should be in proportion to the fall in hematocrit (PCV). In addition, there may be an increase in mean corpuscular volume (MCV) and a decrease in mean corpuscular hemoglobin concentration (MCHC), reflecting the release of larger, less hemoglobinized reticulocytes.

In general, if an adequate reticulocyte response is detected peripherally, then examination of the bone marrow to evaluate the erythroid cell line is unnecessary. In cases of acute hemorrhage or hemolysis, it will take 3 to 4 days until reticulocytosis is detected peripherally. With erythroid hyperplasia accompanying hemorrhage or hemolysis, the maturation sequence in the erythroid line should be orderly, and increased polychromasia should be observed. Very early in a regenerative response, there may be a relative

increase in early erythrocyte precursors, such as rubriblasts and prorubricytes (*Figure 1*). The M:E ratio will depend on the vigor of the erythroid response and may decrease when demand for red cell production is great. Frequently, especially with hemolytic disease, there is concurrent stimulation of production in the myeloid and megakaryocytic cell lines, resulting in a normal M:E ratio. On the CBC, a leukocytosis, consisting of a neutrophilia with left shift and monocytosis, is often seen when there is immune-mediated hemolytic anemia or if hemolysis is associated with an infectious agent.

Granulocytic Hyperplasia

Inflammation that results in a peripheral leukocytosis with a neutrophilia and a left shift will be associated with a hypercellular bone marrow that is due to granulocytic hyperplasia. Early in an inflammatory response or if there is peripheral consumption, the granulocytic hyperplasia may be characterized by a relative increase in the proliferating pool (myeloblasts, promyelocytes, myelocytes) and a depletion of more mature forms (metamyelocytes, bands) (*Figure 2*). This is due to mobilization of cells from the maturation pool. As the inflammatory response becomes more chronic and production is balanced with consumption, an orderly progression of the maturation sequence

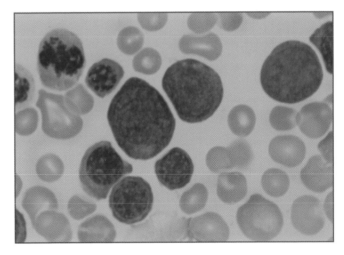

Figure 1. Erythroid hyperplasia in a dog with immune-mediated hemolytic anemia. There is a relative increase in prorubricytes and rubricytes. One mitotic figure in the upper left and polychromasia are seen. Wright's stain, 1000X.

should be re-established. If a cause of inflammation is apparent and the peripheral leukocytosis is regenerative (segmented neutrophils out number bands, which in turn, out number metamyelocytes and myelocytes), then aspiration of the bone marrow is usually unnecessary. Bone marrow evaluation may be needed if a patient has a chronic, unexplained leukocytosis or leukopenia, has a degenerative left shift or disorderly appearance of the peripheral granulocytes, or if intra-marrow infection is suspected.

When granulocyte production is increased, the M:E ratio in the bone marrow will be increased. If the CBC indicates normal red cell mass, then this increase in M:E ratio is primarily due to granulocytic hyperplasia.

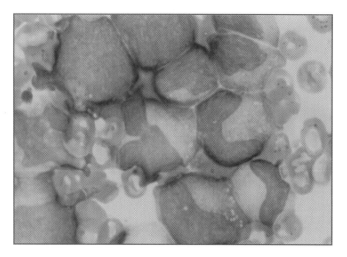

Figure 2. Granulocytic hyperplasia in a dog. There is a relative increase in progranulocytes and myelocytes, and a decrease in band and mature segmented neutrophils (left shift). Wright's stain, 1000X.

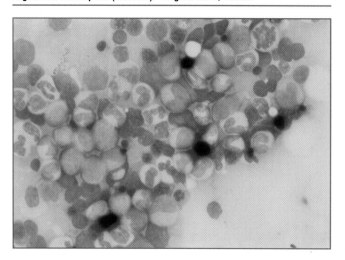

Figure 3. Bone marrow from a dog with granulocytic hyperplasia with a left shift due to inflammation. Anemia of chronic inflammatory disease has developed and is characterized by erythroid hypoplasia and an increase in iron stores, seen as an increase in hemosiderin. Wright's stain, 400X.

Frequently, with chronic inflammation, concurrent erythroid hypoplasia will contribute to the increased M:E ratio, as anemia of chronic disease develops. Anemia of chronic inflammatory disease is the result of sequestration and decreased release of iron from reticuloendothelial stores, making it less available for use by erythrocyte precursors. The CBC will show mild to moderate, normocytic, normochromic, non-regenerative anemia in association with an inflammatory leukogram. In the bone marrow, increased iron stores may be appreciated as an increase in hemosiderin that accompanies the granulocytic hyperplasia (*Figure 3*).

In any case of granulocytic hyperplasia, it is necessary to rule out acute or chronic granulocytic leukemia. In patients with acute granulocytic leukemia, the bone marrow will contain predominantly immature granulocytes, with few mature elements. Distinction of chronic granulocytic leukemia from an inflammatory or leukemoid response is more problematic and is discussed in Chapter 6.

Monocytic/Macrophage Hyperplasia

Hyperplasia of the monocytic cell line in the bone marrow will occur in chronic inflammatory disease or granulomatous disease (*Figure 4*). This should be accompanied by an inflammatory leukogram and a peripheral monocytosis.

Increased numbers of macrophages in the bone marrow may be associated with chronic inflammation, especially with infection with organisms such as *Histoplasma capsulatum, Leishmania infantum*, or *Cytauxzoon felis*. When infection with these organisms is suspected, a bone marrow aspirate may be useful in detecting their presence.

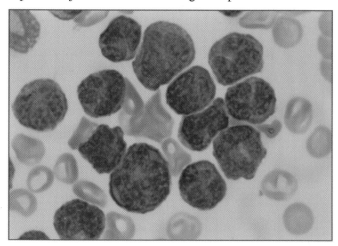

Figure 4. A cluster of monocytic precursors in the bone marrow of a dog. Wright's stain, 1000X.

Increased numbers and activity of macrophages may also be recognized in immune-mediated cytopenias. For example, in the case of immune-mediated hemolytic anemia, increased phagocytosis of red cell precursors may be observed.

Megakaryocytic Hyperplasia

Megakaryocytic hyperplasia may occur whenever there is increased consumption, destruction, or sequestration of platelets that results in increased demand for production of platelets (*Figure 5*). Disorders may include disseminated intravascular coagulation, hemolytic uremic syndrome, other coagulopathies that result in hemorrhage such as rodenticide poisoning or factor deficiencies, immune-mediated thrombocytopenia, or chronic inflammatory disease. Splenomegaly with hypersplenism may result in sequestration of platelets. In general, these syndromes are associated with variable degrees of thrombocytopenia and increases in mean platelet volume may be observed. In the bone marrow, increased numbers of megakaryocytes suggests enhanced thrombopoiesis. An increased proportion of immature megakaryocytes may be seen.

As mentioned above, stimulation of erythroid production may be associated with increased thrombopoiesis, as part of a generalized bone marrow hyperplasia. Additionally, megakaryocytic hyperplasia and thrombocytosis may accompany iron deficiency.

Lymphocytic/Plasma Cell Hyperplasia

Increases in lymphocytes and plasma cells may occur with any disease that results in immune stimulation (*Figure 6*). Infectious agents such as *Ehrlichia canis* are characterized by lymphoplasmacytic hyperplasia. It is necessary to distinguish between an inflammatory process that produces lymphocytic and/or plasmacytic hyperplasia and neoplasms of these cell lines.

Hypoplasia and Aplasia

- ❑ Myelophthisis
- ❑ Aplastic anemia
- ❑ Pure red cell aplasia
- ❑ Secondary marrow suppression

Hypoplastic and Aplastic Conditions

Hypoplasia or aplasia can occur in any cell line in the bone marrow. It is always necessary to rule out extra-marrow causes of suppression of hematopoiesis. This is especially true if there is a cytopenia of only one cell line, while other cell lines are normal to increased in number. If there are cytopenias of more than one cell line, an intra-marrow cause of suppression of hematopoiesis is more likely and a marrow examination should be performed. Myelophthisis or replacement of the marrow by infiltrating neoplastic cells may also result in hypoplasia of hematopoietic precursors. Bone marrow aspirates or core biopsies are useful in

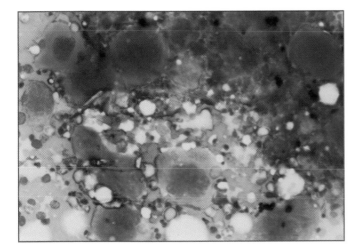

Figure 5. Megakaryocytic hyperplasia in a dog with immune-mediated thrombocytopenia. Particles contain increased numbers of megakaryocytes at various developmental stages. Wright's stain, 200X.

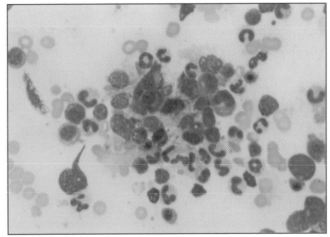

Figure 6. A cluster of well-differentiated plasma cells in the bone marrow of a dog with chronic inflammatory disease. Granulocytic hyperplasia is also evident. Wright's stain, 400X.

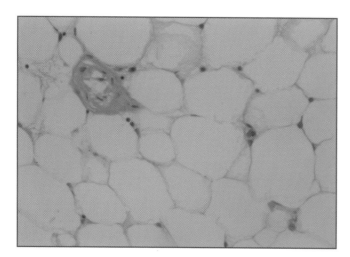

Figure 7. A core biopsy of bone marrow from a dog with aplastic anemia. The bone marrow contains fat and small blood vessels, but no hematopoietic precursors are evident. H&E stain, 200X.

detecting the presence of tumor cells.

Red cell hypoplasia or aplasia will present as a persistent normocytic, normochromic, non-regenerative anemia with a lack of reticulocytosis. Depending on cause, leukocytes and platelets may be normal to increased in numbers. Extra-marrow causes of erythroid hypoplasia include chronic renal disease, hypothyroidism, chronic inflammation or neoplasia, myelotropic viruses such as FeLV, myelotoxic drugs, or prolonged treatment with human recombinant erythropoietin.

Pure red cell aplasia is uncommon in dogs and cats, and erythroid precursors in the bone marrow will be markedly decreased to absent. Pure red cell aplasia may occur in association with infection with FeLV subtype C in cats, and testing for FeLV is warranted in any cat with severe, non-regenerative anemia. Rarely, pure red cell aplasia has been documented in young, FeLV-negative cats. These cats have severe, non-regenerative anemia without punctate reticulo-cytes, have normal leukocyte and platelet counts, and lack organomegaly. In the bone marrow, myeloid and megakaryocytic precursors appear normal, but there is marked erythroid hypoplasia. Some cats also may have a marked lymphocytosis in the bone marrow. These cases appear to respond to long term, aggressive immunosuppressive therapy, suggesting an immune-mediated cause.

Aplastic anemia is characterized by pancytopenia secondary to decreases in hematopoietic progenitors. Unlike myelodysplastic syndromes or myeloproliferative diseases, the bone marrow is hypocellular and may appear either

fatty or fibrotic (*Figure 7*). Bone marrow aspirates may be unsuccessful in these patients and, unless good particles are obtained, may be difficult to distinguish from a hemodiluted sample. Bone marrow core biopsies are often helpful in assessing cellularity in such cases.

Aplastic anemia may be acquired secondary to administration of myelotoxic drugs or infection with myelotropic infectious agents. Infectious agents include FeLV, feline panleukopenia virus, feline immunodeficiency virus (FIV), canine parvovirus, and *E canis*. Hyperestrogenism as a result of iatrogenic administration or endogenous production may cause a pancytopenia. Ten to 20 days following administration of a toxic dose of estrogen, there will be a transient leukocytosis and the marrow will appear hyperplastic. This is followed by progressive cytopenias of all 3 cell lines and hypoplasia of the bone marrow. These changes may be reversible in some patients or may be irreversible and fatally progressive in others. Estrogen-producing neoplasms, such as Sertoli cell or granulosa cell tumors, have also been associated with hypoproliferative cytopenias.

Numerous drugs have been implicated in the production of cytopenias in dogs and cats. Some of these agents are directly myelotoxic while others produce cytopenias as part of an immune response or an idiosyncratic reaction in an individual. Drugs that have been implicated in producing cytopenias in dogs and cats include albendazole, phenobarbital, metronidazole, sulfadiazine, phenylbutazone, meclofenamic acid, fenbendazole, quinidine, griseofulvin, and chloramphenicol. This list is likely to grow as new therapeutic agents are utilized. In addition, radiation therapy and many of the chemotherapeutic agents used for the treatment of cancer, by virtue of their ability to generally affect actively mitotic cells, have the potential to suppress the bone marrow. Careful monitoring of the CBC during therapy is always prudent.

Immune-mediated Diseases

- Immune-mediated hemolytic anemia (IHA)

- Immune-mediated thrombocytopenia (ITP)

Immune-mediated Diseases

Immune-mediated cytopenia occurs in the dog and cat, and most commonly affects erythrocytes and/or platelets. Antibodies are directed at the surface of red blood cells and platelets, resulting in increased phagocytosis and extravascular destruction by macrophages in the spleen and liver. Attachment of complement to the surface of red blood cells also contributes to this process. Partial removal of red cell membrane results in the formation of spherocytes. Occasionally, if appropriate antibodies are produced, complement may be fixed on the surface of erythrocytes and the full attack complex formed, resulting in intravascular hemolysis. In the dog, both immune-mediated hemolytic anemia (IHA) and immune-mediated thrombocytopenia (ITP) occur most frequently in spayed or intact females. While any breed or mixed-breed dog may develop IHA or ITP, there appears to be increased incidence of these syndromes in Cocker Spaniels, Poodles, and Old English Sheep Dogs. While either IHA or ITP may occur alone, in approximately 30% of cases of IHA there is concurrent ITP.

Typically, IHA is associated with a moderate to marked regenerative anemia. Increased release of reticulocytes results in increased polychromasia, macrocytosis, and hypochromasia. Evaluation of the blood film for the presence of spherocytosis or agglutination will aid in diagnosis. Additionally, a Coombs test may be performed. IHA occasionally presents as a non-regenerative anemia. This may occur if the patient is evaluated during the acute stage, prior to the development of a regenerative response. A non-regenerative anemia may also be due to the production of antibodies directed at erythropoietic precursors, effectively inhibiting erythropoiesis. In ITP, thrombocytopenia is usually pronounced (<50,000/µl). Both decreases and increases in mean platelet volume (MPV) have been reported in dogs with ITP and may relate to when the patient is presented. Early in the course of ITP, platelet fragmentation may occur, resulting in a decreased MPV. As the bone marrow responds to the thrombocytopenia, large platelets are released and the MPV will be increased. In patients with either IHA or ITP, a neutrophilia with left shift is usually observed, due to nonspecific bone marrow stimulation. A monocytosis may also be observed in some dogs.

Bone marrow aspirates from patients with either IHA or ITP are hypercellular, with hyperplasia of erythroid,

myeloid, and megakaryocytic lines (*Figure 8*). A reactive histiocytosis consisting of increased numbers of macrophages and increased phagocytosis of either red cell precursors with IHA or platelets with ITP may be observed. With IHA, increased erythrophagocytosis and hemosiderin may be detected. In general, if there is evidence of regeneration in the CBC, bone marrow aspirates are unnecessary in IHA. Bone marrow evaluation should be done in cases of IHA that are nonregenerative. These patients will also show erythroid hyperplasia, however, there may be maturation arrest in the red cell line or increased phagocytosis of early red cell

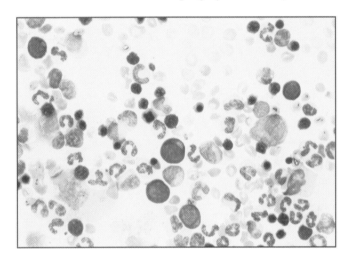

Figure 8. Bone marrow from a dog with immune-mediated hemolytic anemia. There is generalized hyperplasia of the marrow with increases in both erythroid and granulocytic precursors (consequently a normal M:E). The maturation sequences of the hematopoietic precursors are orderly, with many metarubricytes as well as band and segmented neutrophils seen. Wright's stain, 400X.

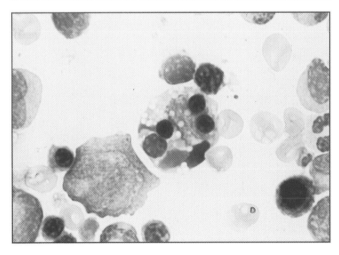

Figure 9. Bone marrow from a dog with IHA illustrating phagocytosis of early red cell precursors by macrophages. Wright's stain, 400X.

precursors (*Figure 9*).

In ITP, normal to increased numbers of megakaryocytes are expected, and there may be relatively more immature megakaryocytes (left shift). However, decreased numbers of megakaryocytes have been reported in up to 20% to 30% of dogs with ITP and may be associated with a poorer prognosis. In some patients, antiplatelet antibody may bind to megakaryocytes, which can be demonstrated by immunofluorescence.

IHA and ITP usually are initially treated with corticosteroids. Occasional cases may prove refractory and require more aggressive immunosuppressive therapy. Vincristine (Oncovin®, Eli Lilly, Indianapolis, IN) has been used in patients with ITP to increase platelet numbers. Vincristine is a vinca alkaloid that interferes with the formation of the mitotic spindle in cells that are actively dividing. Treatment of dogs with ITP usually results in an increase in platelet numbers within 1 week. It is important to note that vincristine therapy is associated with production of dysplastic changes in hematopoietic precursors within the bone marrow. These effects may be seen within hours of initiation of vincristine therapy and consist primarily of abnormalities in the red cell line. Morphologic alterations include increased numbers of mitotic figures, fragmentation of nuclei, and abnormal nuclear configurations. Mild dysplastic changes may also be seen in nonerythroid precursors, however, these tend to be less common. Awareness of potential effects of a chemotherapeutic agent on hematopoietic precursors is important when considering evaluation of bone marrow once therapy has begun.

Inflammatory Disease

The appearance of the bone marrow during inflammatory disease will depend on the stage at which the bone marrow is examined. Acute inflammation may be associated with a depletion of the storage pool of granulocytes, resulting in an apparent left shift in granulopoiesis. As the inflammatory process becomes more prolonged, granulocytic hyperplasia often occurs with an increase in the M:E ratio and a more orderly appearance to the maturation sequence. With severe inflammatory disease, toxic changes in granulocytic precursors may be evident (*Figure 10*). These include cytoplasmic vacuolization, cytoplasmic basophilia and the presence of Döhle bodies. If toxicity is severe, cytoplasmic vacuoles and altered cytoplasmic maturation may be observed in other cells lines as well.

As inflammation becomes chronic, anemia frequently develops, resulting in erythroid hypoplasia and increased hemosiderin deposits. This will further exaggerate the increase in M:E ratio. With chronic inflammation or with development of granulomatous disease, there will be increased demand for and production of monocytes. Within the bone marrow, macrophages may increase in number and become more actively phagocytic. With chronic antigenic stimulation, lymphocytes and plasma cells will also increase in numbers.

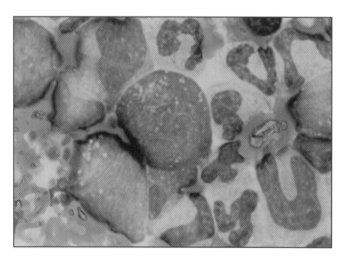

Figure 10. Bone marrow from a dog with inflammatory disease. Cytoplasmic vacuolation is seen as part of toxic changes in the granulocytic precursors. Wright's stain, 1000X.

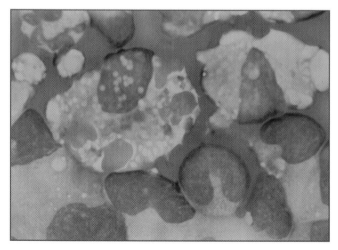

Figure 11. Histiocytic hyperplasia with marked erythrophagocytosis present in a dog with hemophagocytic syndrome. Two morphologically normal macrophages are seen, one of which contains phagocytized RBCs and hemosiderin. In addition, there is granulocytic hyperplasia, compatible with inflammatory disease. Wright's stain, 1000X.

Hemophagocytic syndrome or hemophagocytic histiocytosis has been observed in dogs and cats and is characterized by macrophage proliferation secondary to infectious, metabolic or neoplastic diseases. This macrophage proliferation occurs primarily in the bone marrow, however, spleen, liver, and lymph nodes may also be affected. Clinical signs are variable and dependent on the inciting condition. The CBC from affected individuals is characterized by peripheral cytopenias involving 2 or more cells lines, the presence of red blood cell fragments, and, occasionally, activated monocytes. The bone marrow may be hypocellular to hypercellular, with variable infiltration of macrophages. A prominent feature of this syndrome is pronounced erythrophagocytosis (*Figure 11*). The increase in phagocytosis of red cell precursors appears to be due to inappropriate activation of macrophages as part of an inflammatory response. In contrast to neoplastic proliferation of histiocytes, the macrophages of hemophagocytic syndrome are normal in appearance. Hemophagocytic syndrome usually resolves with successful treatment of the primary disease.

Infectious Diseases

Infectious agents are uncommonly detected in bone marrow aspirates. However, for some infectious diseases, such as leishmaniasis, histoplasmosis, and cytauxzoonosis, a bone marrow aspirate may be helpful in making a diagnosis.

Bacterial infections
Mycobacteria

Although bacteria are rarely detected in bone marrow aspirates, evaluation of bone marrow aspirates occasionally has been used to diagnose mycobacterial infections in animals with disseminated disease. *Mycobacteria* species are non-spore-forming, straight to slightly curved, pleomorphic bacilli that may be associated with localized cutaneous or disseminated disease. Pathogenic species infecting dogs and cats include *Mycobacteria tuberculosis, M bovis, M avium* complex, *M lepraemurium*, and various other opportunistic species. *Mycobacteria* organisms have a high lipid content in the cell wall, which enables them to retain carbofuchsin stains after treatment with acid or alcohol, and thus mycobacteria are called acid-fast organisms. The high lipid content also prevents *Mycobacteria* organisms from staining with routine cytologic stains. In cytologic preparations, the organisms appear as unstained rods, 0.2 to 0.5 microns

wide and 1.0 to 3.0 microns long (*Figure 12*). Organisms appear extracellular or intracellular, usually within macrophages, which often are numerous. Acid-fast staining is recommended for presumptive diagnosis. Definitive diagnosis is based on culture and classification, which often takes 4 to 6 weeks. Recently, polymerase chain reaction technology has been used on clinical specimens to more rapidly detect *Mycobacteria* species.

Rickettsial infections
Ehrlichia

Ehrlichia species are obligate, intracellular rickettsial parasites that cause systemic disease. The organisms are transmitted by ticks and primarily infect dogs. Only rare, isolated cases have been described in cats, and the species that infect cats after natural exposure have not been determined. Several *Ehrlichia* species have been associated with disease in dogs. These include *Ehrlichia canis, E chaffeensis, E*

Infectious Diseases

❏ Bacterial infections
  Mycobacteria

❏ Rickettsial infections
  Ehrlichia

❏ Protozoal infections
  Leishmaniasis
  Cytauxzoonosis
  Babesiosis

❏ Mycoplasma-like infections
  Haemobartonellosis

❏ Fungal infections
  Histoplasmosis

❏ Viral infections
  Parvovirus
  Distemper virus
  Feline leukemia virus (FeLV)
  Feline immunodeficiency virus (FIV)

risticii, E ewingii, E equi, E phagocytophilia, and *E platys*. The cell type infected and the spectrum of clinical signs depends on the species of Ehrlichia. Most information about pathogenesis and clinical findings is related to *E canis* infection.

E canis infects monocytes and causes multisystemic clinical signs including anorexia, depression, lethargy, weight loss, and bleeding diatheses. *E canis* infection also has been associated with anterior uveitis, retinal disease, neurologic abnormalities and polyarthritis. Infected dogs may have lymphadenomegaly and splenomegaly. Laboratory abnormalities include nonregenerative anemia, leukopenia, thrombocytopenia, and hypergammaglobulinemia. Bone marrow hypoplasia with plasma cell hyperplasia occurs in the severe, chronic phase of the disease.

The diagnosis of ehrlichiosis usually is made based on clinical signs, hematologic abnormalities, and serologic findings. Recently, immunoblotting and PCR have been used to distinguish among the different *Ehrlichia* species. *Ehrlichia* organisms usually are not easily detected by routine light microscopy. Occasionally, the intracytoplasmic inclusions called morula may be seen in bone marrow aspirates from dogs with *E canis* infection. Morula appear as light blue or purple, slightly granular, round to oval structures, 2.0 to 6.0 microns in diameter. Ultrastructurally, morula contain numerous membrane-bound organisms, which likely impart the granular appearance to the morula at the light microscopic level.

Protozoal infections
Leishmaniasis

Leishmaniasis is a chronic, systemic disease caused by protozoan parasites of the genus *Leishmania*. Leishmaniasis is rarely recognized in the US and most dogs in which it is reported have been imported or have traveled to parts of the world in which the disease is endemic. However, autochthonous foci of Leishmaniasis have been reported in Ohio, Oklahoma, and Texas. Cats are only rarely infected, even in endemic areas. Clinical findings in dogs with leishmaniasis are variable and include weight loss, somnolence, and exercise intolerance. Lymphadenomegaly and cutaneous involvement occur in the majority of dogs with leishmaniasis.

The most common organism associated with disease in dogs is *Leishmania infantum*. The parasite is transmitted by blood-sucking sandflies. The nonflagellated form of the parasite, called an amastigote, replicates by binary fission within macrophages. The amastigote is ovoid to round, 2.5 to 5.0 microns long and 1.5 to 2.0 microns wide, and contains a reddish nucleus and a characteristic purple, rod-shaped kinetoplast (*Figure 13*). Definitive diagnosis can be made by identifying the organism in macrophages from lymph node or bone marrow aspirates. Various immunodiagnostic tests also are available and PCR detection of leishmanial DNA in bone marrow recently has been described.

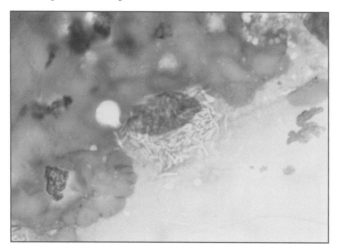

Figure 12. *Mycobacteria* organisms from a dog with systemic infection. The organisms appear as unstained rods, 0.2 to 0.5 microns wide and 1.0 to 3.0 microns long, and most often are located within macrophages. Acid-fast staining is recommended for presumptive diagnosis. Wright's stain, 1000X.

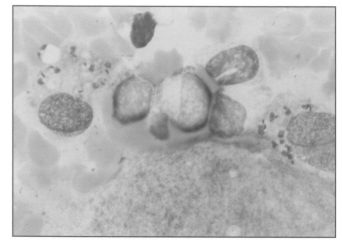

Figure 13. Two macrophages with intracellular *Leishmania* organisms from a dog with systemic Leishmaniasis. This dog had traveled to Greece, which is an endemic area. The amastigote stage of the organism is oval to round, 2.5 to 5.0 microns long and 1.5 to 2.0 microns wide. A roundish nucleus and a characteristic rod-shaped kinetoplast typically are present. Wright's stain, 1000X.

Cytauxzoonosis

Cytauxzoonosis is a protozoal disease of domestic and exotic cats that occurs in several south central and southeastern states in the US. The North American bobcat appears to be the natural reservoir host. The sporadic occurrence, short course of illness, and usually fatal nature of the disease suggest that the domestic cat is an incidental dead-end host. Clinical findings include fever or subnormal temperature, anorexia, dyspnea, lethargy, dark urine, dehydration, depression icterus, and pallor. Most cats die within 5 days of onset of clinical signs.

The etiologic agent of cytauxzoonosis is *Cytauxzoon felis*, a protozoan parasite transmitted by ticks. There is a tissue phase and an erythrocytic phase of parasite development in cats. The tissue phase involves schizogony within macrophages. Infected macrophages line the lumen of veins in most organs, which can result in vascular occlusion and ischemic necrosis. Infected macrophages containing schizonts can be found in tissue aspirates from the bone marrow, spleen, or lymph node, or sometimes are seen on the feathered edge of peripheral blood smears (*Figure 14*). The merozoite stage of the organism develops within infected macrophages, is released from macrophages, and invades erythrocytes. Parasitized erythrocytes are observed late in the disease, usually during a febrile episode. *Cytauxzoon* organisms (piroplasts) in erythrocytes are round, "signet-ring" structures; bipolar, oval forms; tetrad forms; or round dots ranging in size from 0.5 to 2.0 microns in diameter. The cytoplasm stains light blue and the nucleus is dark red or purple.

Babesiosis

Canine babesiosis is a tick-transmitted disease caused by either *Babesia canis* or *B gibsoni*. It occurs worldwide, but in the US the disease is most common along the Gulf Coast and in the south, central, and southwestern states. No cases of feline babesiosis have been reported in the US. Canine babesiosis may be associated with acute hemolytic anemia or peracute, hypotensive shock and multiple-organ dysfunction. Clinical presentation varies with age and breed, species of parasite, and geographic location. Acute disease is more common and is characterized by anorexia, hemolytic anemia, thrombocytopenia, lymphadenomegaly, and splenomegaly. Leukocyte abnormalities are less consistent but may include leukocytosis, neutrophilia, neutropenia, lymphocytosis, and eosinophilia.

Babesia canis is a piriform-shaped organism (2.4 microns × 5.0 microns) that occurs singly or in pairs in erythrocytes. *B gibsoni* is much smaller (1.0 microns × 3.2 microns), more pleomorphic, and usually occurs as a single intraerythrocytic organism. Definitive diagnosis is made by demonstrating organisms within infected erythrocytes or by positive serology. Only small numbers of parasites may be present on peripheral blood smears. Parasitized erythrocytes also may be seen in splenic impression smears and bone marrow aspirates (*Figure 15*).

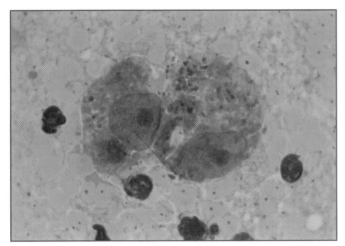

Figure 14. Macrophage containing a schizont of *Cytauxzoon felis*. Infected macrophages can be found in aspirates from bone marrow, spleen, or lymph nodes. The piroplast stage may be seen in the RBCs in peripheral blood. Wright's stain, 1000X.

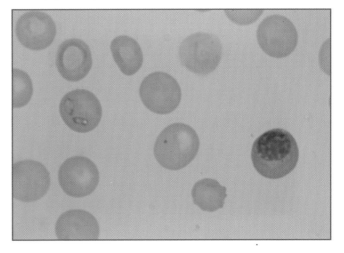

Figure 15. A RBC with 2 piriform-shaped *Babesia canis* organisms. Parasitized erythrocytes may be seen in peripheral blood and in tissue aspirates from the bone marrow or spleen. Wright's stain, 1000X.

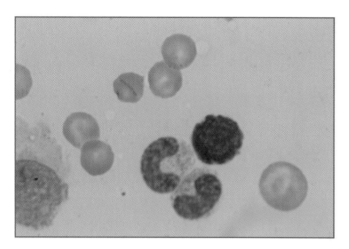

Figure 16. A RBC with a chain of *Haemobartonella* organisms is shown in the center left. *H canis* more often forms chains of organisms than does *H felis*. Wright's stain, 1000X.

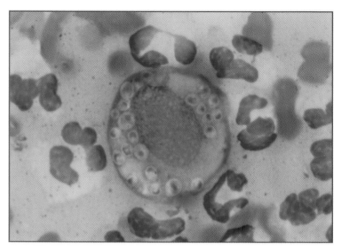

Figure 17. A macrophage with numerous intracellular *Histoplasma* organisms from a cat with systemic infection. The organisms are 2.0 to 4.0 microns in diameter and have a basophilic center with a light halo. Wright's stain, 1000X.

Mycoplasma-like infections
Haemobartonellosis

Haemobartonellosis is caused by *Haemobartonella felis* in cats and *H canis* in dogs. The organism is an epicellular erythrocytic parasite that is associated with hemolytic anemia. On Romanowsky-stained blood films, *Haemobartonella* organisms appear as blue-staining rods, cocci, or ring-shaped structures, 0.5 microns in diameter. *H canis* more commonly forms chains across the surface of erythrocytes than does *H felis*. Parasitemia is cyclical and few, if any, parasites may be seen in blood films for several days following parasitemia. Moderate to marked fluctuations in PCV may be associated with parasitemic episodes. The anemia usually is regenerative. Marked erythroid hyperplasia and erythrophagocytosis often are present on bone marrow aspirates. Although most often detected in peripheral blood, organisms also may be present in bone marrow aspirates (*Figure 16*).

Haemobartonella felis likely will be reclassified from a rickettsial-like organism to a mycoplasma organism, based on recent nucleotide sequencing. It also is likely that *H canis* will be reclassified as a mycoplasma organism, if RNA sequencing data are similar to that described for *H felis*. RNA sequencing has also led to the development of polymerase chain reaction based assays for detection of Haemobartonella organisms. This should greatly increase the recognition of infected animals.

Fungal infections
Histoplasmosis

Histoplasmosis occurs in dogs and cats and is caused by the dimorphic fungus, *Histoplasma capsulatum*. Although the organism has been isolated from the soil in many states, the disease occurs most commonly in the region of the Ohio, Missouri, and Mississippi Rivers. Inhaled microconidia convert to the yeast stage in the lung, and are phagocytized by macrophages. The disease may be localized to the lung or there may be lymphatic or hematogenous dissemination. The GI tract also may be a primary site of infection.

Clinical findings are variable and may include depression, weight loss, fever, anorexia, dyspnea, tachypnea, peripheral or visceral lymphadenomegaly, splenomegaly, and hepatomegaly. In dogs with histoplasmosis involving the GI tract, there may be signs associated with large-bowel diarrhea. Laboratory abnormalities include normocytic, normochromic non-regenerative anemia, likely related to anemia of chronic inflammatory disease. There also may be *Histoplasma* infection of the bone marrow, in which case the yeast organisms may be demonstrated within bone marrow macrophages. Routine hematologic stains can be used to demonstrate *Histoplasma* organisms, which appear as small (2.0 -4.0 microns in diameter) round structures with a basophilic center and a lighter halo (*Figure 17*). The halo is caused by shrinkage of the organisms during staining. In most infected tissues, numerous organisms are present within macrophages. Occasionally, budding organisms may be present.

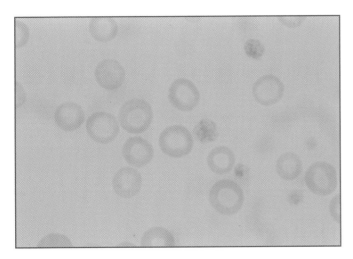

Figure 18. Blood film from a dog with iron deficiency is characterized by anisocytosis and marked hypochromasia. Wright's stain, 1000X.

Viral infections
Parvovirus

There are several viral infections that may affect the bone marrow. Cats infected with panleukopenia virus develop marked leukopenia from neutropenia and lymphopenia because of depressed myelopoiesis. In protracted cases, there may be inhibition of erythropoiesis and megakaryocytopoiesis. Dogs with parvovirus infection also develop marked leukopenia from neutropenia and lymphopenia. As granulopoiesis is reestablished during convalescence, there may be giant forms of neutrophils with bizarre nuclear morphology. More normal appearing neutrophils usually are present within a couple of days.

Distemper virus

In dogs with distemper virus infection, there may be inclusions in immature erythrocytes and leukocytes in the blood and bone marrow. Inclusions in erythrocytes are round to oval, 0.5 to 3.0 microns in diameter, and stain light blue to gray. These inclusions appear to be aggregates of paramyxovirus-like nucleocapsids.

Feline leukemia virus

Numerous neoplastic and non-neoplastic diseases have been associated with feline leukemia virus (FeLV) infection in cats. Hematologic diseases include lymphoid and myeloid malignancies, immunodeficiency, secondary bacterial infections, regenerative and non-regenerative or aplastic anemia, thrombocytopenia, pancytopenia, panleukopenia-

like syndrome, cyclic hematopoiesis, and thymic atrophy. Bone marrow findings vary, depending on what disease has developed. FeLV-induced hematopoietic neoplasia is discussed in further detail in a later section.

Feline immunodeficiency virus

Cats with asymptomatic, naturally-acquired feline immunodeficiency virus (FIV) infection rarely have hematologic abnormalities. However, some cats with FIV-associated illnesses have peripheral blood cytopenias that may be accompanied by subtle morphologic abnormalities in the bone marrow. Morphologic abnormalities in the bone marrow include myeloid hyperplasia, erythroid hyperplasia, megakaryocytic hyperplasia, mild megaloblastic changes in erythroid cells, increased numbers of lymphocytes and plasma cells, and infiltration with neoplastic lymphoid cells.

Metabolic Diseases

❑ Iron deficiency
❑ Vitamin B_{12}/folate deficiency

Metabolic diseases
Iron deficiency

Depending on the stage of disease, patients with iron deficiency will present with a normocytic normochromic to microcytic hypochromic anemia (*Figure 18*). Because iron deficiency is usually due to chronic blood loss in adult animals, polychromasia may be seen, but the anemia will become nonregenerative as iron depletion progresses. The bone marrow of patients with iron deficiency will vary in cellularity. Frequently samples appear hypercellular with a relative increase in the proportion of early erythroid precursors or a left shift in the erythroid line (*Figure 19*). As iron deficiency becomes fully developed, asynchrony of nuclear and cytoplasmic maturation may occur resulting in production and release of microcytic hypochromic red cells. There may be an increase in ineffective erythropoiesis, suggested by an increase in phagocytosis of red cell precursors by macrophages. Thrombocytosis and megakaryocytic hyperplasia often accompany iron deficiency anemia. Bone marrow iron stores will be markedly decreased to absent and hemosiderin will not be apparent in bone marrow aspi-

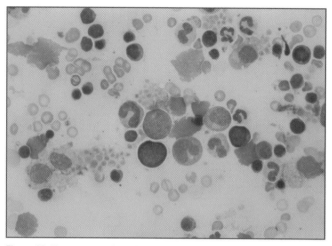

Figure 19. Bone marrow from the same dog with iron deficiency. There are decreased numbers of metarubricytes and a relative increase in rubricytes. Some asynchrony in nuclear and cytoplasmic maturation is evident with clumping of chromatin out pacing hemoglobinization of the cells. Wright's stain, 1000X.

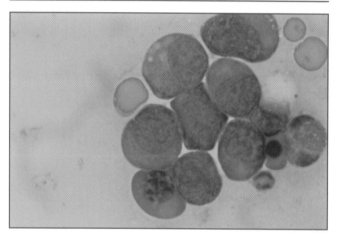

Figure 20. Megaloblastic changes observed in the bone marrow from a cat with myelodysplastic disease secondary to FeLV infection. There is asynchrony of nuclear and cytoplasmic maturation evident within the red cell precursors, which contain large, immature nuclei with fine chromatin and nucleoli, but hemoglobinized and granular cytoplasm. Wright's stain, 1000X.

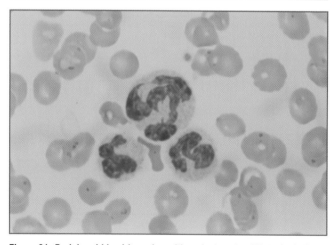

Figure 21. Peripheral blood from dog with a giant neutrophil, typical of megaloblastic changes affecting the myeloid precursors. Wright's stain, 1000X.

rate smears. It is best to evaluate bone marrow iron stores using a special stain for iron, such as Prussian blue. Often, however, bone marrow changes with iron deficiency are not distinctive. As further evidence of iron deficiency, decreases in serum ferritin, serum iron, and percent transferrin saturation may be detected.

Megaloblastic anemia and vitamin B$_{12}$ and folate deficiency

Deficiency of either vitamin B$_{12}$ or folate may result in megaloblastic changes within the bone marrow. While marrow aspirates from affected individuals are cellular, there is asynchrony of cytoplasmic and nuclear maturation in the erythroid line, resulting in a maturation arrest at the prorubricyte and basophilic rubricyte stages. Because deficiency of vitamin B$_{12}$ or folate affects synthesis of DNA, there is interference with mitosis and the progressive condensation of nuclear chromatin normally observed in red cell precursors. Hemoglobinization is unimpaired. Typically, red cell precursors contain a large, immature-appearing nucleus with fine, unclumped chromatin in association with more mature, hemoglobinized cytoplasm (*Figure 20*). In dogs and cats, anemias proven responsive to vitamin B$_{12}$ or folate therapy are usually normocytic; however, macrocytic red cells may be released. Maturation arrest may also be observed in myeloid and megakaryocytic precursors. Hypersegmented and giant neutrophils, with or without neutropenia, may be present (*Figure 21*). Megakaryocytes may have fewer nuclei, and platelets may show more variation in size.

It is nearly impossible to produce a dietary deficiency of vitamin B$_{12}$ or folate in dogs and cats, especially if they are kept on a commercial diet. However, an inherited deficiency of the intestinal receptor for vitamin B$_{12}$ has been documented in Giant Schnauzer dogs, resulting in malabsorption of this nutrient and subsequent megaloblastic changes in the bone marrow. Other diseases that cause intestinal malabsorption have the potential to cause deficiency states. Treatments with drugs that interfere with folate metabolism such as sulfonamides, phenytoin, aminopterin, or methotrexate, also have the potential to affect folate availability for hematopoiesis. Again, however, these effects tend to be very rare in dogs and cats. Megaloblastic changes that are unrelated to vitamin deficiency and unresponsive to vitamin supplementation are observed in some normal poodles and in cats with FeLV-related myeloproliferative disease.

Congenital Diseases
Cyclic hematopoiesis (cyclic neutropenia)

A syndrome of cyclic fluctuations in blood cell counts has been described in Collie dogs with a grey coat color. Most notable is the development of severe neutropenia (<1,000/µl) with concurrent reticulocytosis which takes place with a periodicity of approximately 12 days. A thrombocytosis occurs several days prior to the neutropenic nadir and a monocytosis peaks as the neutropenia resolves. These dogs tend to be anemic despite periodic increases in reticulocyte counts, but fluctuations in red cell numbers are not apparent due to the long life span of these cells in circulation. Bone marrow aspirates from these dogs are cellular, but periodically show maturation arrest in the myeloid proliferation pool and lack of mature neutrophils. In addition to cycling of cell number, there also appear to be functional defects in neutrophils and platelets from these animals. Grey Collies with cyclic hematopoiesis have increased susceptibility to infection.

Cyclic hematopoiesis of grey Collies is an autosomal recessive inherited disorder that appears to be due to a regulatory defect in early hematopoietic stem cells. Peripheral neutrophil counts and hematopoiesis can be maintained by administration of G-CSF or SCF, suggesting that altered stem cell responsiveness to these growth factors plays a role in the pathogenesis of this syndrome.

A similar phenomenon of cyclic neutropenia has been reported in several cats infected with FeLV. Neutropenic cycles in these cats occurred every 8 to 14 days and resolution of neutropenia was preceded by a monocytosis. Bone marrow aspirates from these cats showed a predominance of progranulocytes during the neutropenic episodes. During periods with normal neutrophil counts, myeloid hyperplasia with segmented neutrophils was observed in the bone marrow.

Pelger-Huët syndrome

Pelger-Huët syndrome has been reported in dogs and cats. It is an inherited disorder in which the nuclei of granulocytes fail to undergo normal segmentation during the maturation process. Typical Pelger-Huët cells have oval to bean-shaped nuclei, with mature-appearing, clumped chro-

Congenital Diseases

☐ Cyclic hematopoiesis (cyclic neutropenia)

☐ Pelger-Huët syndrome

☐ Chédiak-Higashi syndrome

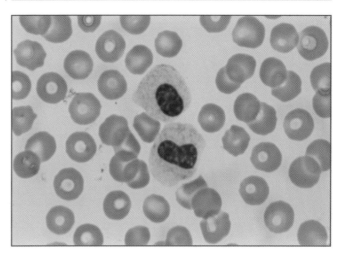

Figure 22. Blood film from a dog with Pelger-Huët syndrome. The 2 neutrophils have non-segmented, oval to bean-shaped nuclei with mature-appearing chromatin and mature cytoplasm. Wright's stain, 1000X.

matin (*Figure 22*). Neutrophils from affected dogs and cats function normally, and there does not appear to be any health consequences of this condition. Usually, this anomaly is detected as an incidental finding during examination of a CBC as part of a routine physical or when the patient is being evaluated for another condition. As such, a bone marrow examination is unnecessary, but would have the appearance of a maturation arrest at the level of myelocytes and metamyelocytes. A pseudo-Pelger-Huët appearance of neutrophils can occur as an acquired change due to dysmyelopoiesis secondary to severe infection. Neutrophils from patients with infection may also display toxic changes such as cytoplasmic basophilia, vacuolization, and Döhle bodies. To distinguish a true from a pseudo-Pelger-Huët case it is necessary to rule out infection and to repeat the CBC to ascertain that the condition does not resolve with time. Pelger-Huët syndrome must also be distinguished from myelogenous leukemia.

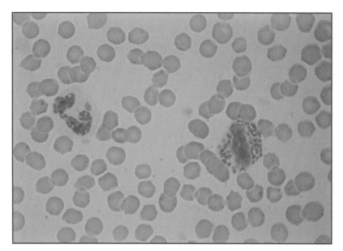

Figure 23. Blood film from a Persian cat with Chédiak-Higashi syndrome. The neutrophil contains 2 pink, cytoplasmic inclusions, typical of giant lysosomes. The granules of the eosinophil are enlarged and abnormally shaped. Wright's stain, 1000X. (Blood film courtesy of Dr. Mary Anna Thrall.)

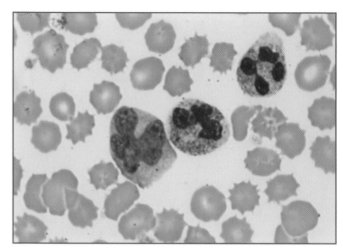

Figure 24. Blood film from a dog with mucopolysaccharidosis VI. There are prominent, purple-staining granules (Alder-Reilly bodies) in the neutrophils. Wright's stain, 1000X. (Blood film courtesy of Dr. Sharon Dial.)

Chédiak-Higashi syndrome

Chédiak-Higashi syndrome is an inherited, autosomal recessive disorder that has been reported in Persian cats. This defect results in abnormal formation of giant lysosomes, which may be detected as large, pink staining inclusions in granulocytes (*Figure 23*). Episodes of neutropenia are frequently observed and are responsive to treatment with G-CSF. In addition, neutrophils show functional defects. As a result, patients with Chédiak-Higashi syndrome may have increased susceptibility to infection. Platelets from cats with Chédiak-Higashi syndrome lack dense bodies and have functional defects, resulting in a bleeding tendency. Because the formation of melanin granules is also abnormal in this condition, Persian cats with Chédiak-Higashi syndrome show color dilution of the fur and eyes (blue smoke hair color and yellow eyes). This condition is usually diagnosed by finding typical morphologic features in the granulocytes on a blood film. These same features will be apparent on bone marrow aspirates.

Lysosomal Storage Diseases

❑ Mucopolysaccharidosis VI

❑ α-mannosidosis

Lysosomal Storage Diseases

A number of lysosomal storage diseases have been reported in dogs and cats. Typically, these conditions are diagnosed as the result of physical examination and findings of typical morphologic changes in cells in the peripheral blood. For example, mucopolysaccharidosis VI in cats and dogs is characterized by the presence of metachromatic granules (Alder-Reilly bodies) in the cytoplasm of neutrophils, eosinophils, lymphocytes and monocytes (*Figure 24*). Cytoplasmic vacuoles in lymphocytes and monocytes are typically seen in cats with α-mannosidosis. While similar inclusions are found in the hematopoietic cells, bone marrow aspirates are usually unremarkable and not routinely performed, unless bone marrow transplantation is used as a therapeutic measure. Confirmation of the metabolic defect is done using specific biochemical tests.

Chapter 6: **Hematopoietic Neoplasia**

Hematopoietic neoplasia involves transformation and clonal expansion of hematopoietic stem cells, lymphoid cells, or myeloid cells. Neoplastic and dysplastic processes involving lymphoid or myeloid cells are referred to as lymphoproliferative or myeloproliferative disorders, respectively. Neoplastic transformation of lymphoid cells results in lymphoma, multiple myeloma, plasma cell tumors, or lymphoid leukemia, whereas neoplastic transformation of myeloid cells results in myeloid leukemia.

Lymphoid neoplasia is more common than myeloid neoplasia in dogs and cats and lymphoma is the most common lymphoid neoplasm. Lymphoma initially involves tissues other than the bone marrow, but bone marrow infiltration may occur in late stage disease. This is in contrast to lymphoid and myeloid leukemia, which originate in the bone marrow. The etiology of hematopoietic neoplasia in dogs is unknown. There is a direct association between feline leukemia virus (FeLV) infection and hematopoietic neoplasia in cats.

Bone marrow evaluation often is useful in the diagnosis of hematopoietic neoplasia. In lymphoma, bone marrow aspirates may be used in clinical staging schemes, as a diagnostic aid in animals with hypercalcemia, or in supporting a diagnosis of lymphoma in animals with atypical clinical signs or tissue involvement. A bone marrow aspirate often is very important in establishing a definitive diagnosis of lymphoid or myeloid leukemia and multiple myeloma.

Abnormal proliferation and maturation of neoplastic hematopoietic cells are expressed as increases in cell number and abnormal cell morphology. In some cases, multiple cell types may be affected and there may be transition from one cell type to another in the same individual. In most cases, however, one cell type predominates and the hematopoietic neoplasm is classified based on that cell type. In addition to proliferation of the neoplastic clone, there often is decreased proliferation of other hematopoietic cells, resulting in peripheral blood cytopenias of non-neoplastic cell types. In some cases, peripheral blood cytopenias are the first abnormality recognized, and may be an indication for a bone marrow aspirate to pursue a diagnosis of hematopoietic neoplasia. The term myelophthisis is some-times used when the bone marrow is infiltrated with neoplastic (or inflammatory) cells, resulting in a marked decrease or absence of normal hematopoietic cells.

Lymphoproliferative Disorders

- ❏ Lymphoma
- ❏ Multiple myeloma
- ❏ Plasma cell tumors
- ❏ Leukemia
  - Acute lymphoblastic leukemia (ALL)
  - Chronic lymphocytic leukemia (CLL)

Lymphoproliferative Disorders
Lymphoma

Lymphoma (malignant lymphoma, lymphosarcoma) refers to the malignant transformation of lymphoid cells that originates in tissues other than the bone marrow. Lymphoma is the most common type of hematopoietic neoplasm in dogs and cats. Based on tissue distribution, several anatomic forms have been recognized. These include multicentric, alimentary, thymic, and cutaneous lymphoma. The most common form of lymphoma in dogs is multicentric, which typically is a disease of dogs greater than 5 years of age. Golden Retrievers, Boxers, Basset Hounds, Saint Bernards, and Scottish Terriers are among the breeds at increased risk for lymphoma. The etiology of lymphoma in dogs is unknown. Recent studies have documented a shift in the traditional signalment and anatomic form in cats with lymphoma. Previously, cats with lymphoma had a median age of 4 to 6 years, a 60% to 70% incidence of FeLV antigenemia, and mediastinal lymphoma as the most common form. Current data suggest that the median age is 9.5 years, only 25% are FeLV positive, and the most common form is alimentary lymphoma.

Clinical findings associated with lymphoma are variable and reflect the organs and tissues infiltrated and the extent of involvement. Dogs with multicentric lymphoma often are presented because of nonpainful enlargement of multiple peripheral lymph nodes. Clinical signs associated with the alimentary form include anorexia, weight loss, vomiting, and diarrhea. With lymphoma involving the thymus or mediastinal lymph nodes, there may be dyspnea, tachypnea, regurgitation, coughing, and pleural effusion. A clinical staging scheme based on tissue distribution has been developed for dogs with lymphoma. This has been useful in establishing prognoses and designing chemotherapy protocols. Bone marrow involvement indicates stage V lymphoma, which has a worse prognosis than the other stages.

Laboratory changes often are unremarkable. There may be non-regenerative anemia and circulation of neoplastic lymphocytes. Although as many as 50% of dogs with lymphoma may have circulating neoplastic lymphocytes, the number of circulating neoplastic cells may be so low that they are easily missed on routine evaluation. Hypercalcemia occurs in some dogs with lymphoma, especially if there is mediastinal involvement. Hypercalcemia in cats with lymphoma is less common.

The degree of differentiation and neoplastic cell type may affect response to treatment and prognosis in dogs and cats with lymphoma. Histologic classification schemes have been developed for canine lymphoma and are based on evaluation of tissue architecture, cell morphology, and mitotic rate in formalin-fixed sections. Cytologic classification is based almost entirely on nuclear characteristics, including nuclear size, shape, and chromatin pattern and nucleolar number and size. A similar classification scheme has not been developed for cats.

It may be more clinically useful to classify lymphoma based on the lineage of neoplastic lymphocytes. Immunophenotyping can be performed to determine if neoplastic lymphocytes are B or T lineage, which cannot be determined by morphologic features. B lymphocytes are positive for CD19, CD20, or CD21 (*See Chapter 4, Table 2*). Staining for surface immunoglobulin also can be used to identify B lymphocytes. T lymphocytes are positive for CD3 and either CD4 or CD8. Most multicentric lymphomas in dogs involve B lymphocytes, but involvement of T lymphocytes has been reported. Thymic lymphoma in dogs and cats involves T lymphocytes. FeLV-induced lym-

phoma usually involves T lymphocytes. Alimentary lymphoma most often occurs in FeLV-negative cats and usually involves B lymphocytes. In cats with FIV-induced lymphoma, the neoplastic lymphocytes most commonly are B lymphocytes. Results of immunophenotyping suggest that dogs with T-cell lymphoma have a worse prognosis than dogs with B-cell lymphoma, but this does not appear to be true in cats.

The diagnosis of lymphoma involving the bone marrow is based on the detection of neoplastic lymphocytes in bone marrow aspirates or core biopsies. The number of neoplastic lymphocytes detected in bone marrow aspirates is variable and the number necessary for a diagnosis of lymphoma has not been clearly established. Typically, greater than 30% of all nucleated cells in the bone marrow are neoplastic lymphocytes in dogs and cats with lymphoma. This is in contrast to less than 10% and 15% mature, small lymphocytes in the bone marrow from healthy dogs and cats, respectively.

In most cases, the neoplastic lymphoid cells appear immature and are easily distinguished from normal small lymphocytes. Normal small lymphocytes are smaller than a neutrophil and have condensed chromatin, inconspicuous nucleoli, and a very narrow rim of cytoplasm. Neoplastic lymphoid cells are the same size as or larger than a neutrophil, and often have a moderate amount of basophilic cytoplasm. Nuclei are large and usually are round, but indented or irregular nuclear shapes may occur. The chromatin often is finely granular and multiple, prominent nucleoli of variable size typically are present (*Figure 1*). In some cases, however, the chromatin is moderately clumped and nucleoli are absent. The cytoplasm sometimes contains vacuoles, but the significance of these is not known (*Figure 2*). In some cases, azurophilic cytoplasmic granules may be present, which suggests that the cells are a subset of T lymphocytes or NK cells called granular lymphocytes (*Figure 3*). The clinical relevance of this cell type in dogs and cats with lymphoma has not been determined.

When large numbers of morphologically immature lymphoid cells are present, the diagnosis of bone marrow infiltration by neoplastic cells is relatively straightforward. However, it may be difficult to distinguish between neoplastic lymphocytes from Stage V lymphoma and acute lymphoid leukemia based on morphology. In general, dogs with lymphoma have marked lymphadenomegaly and few

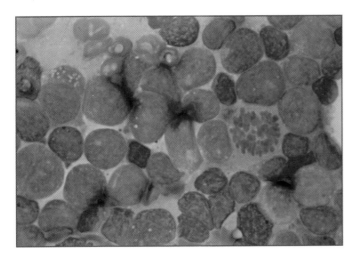

Figure 1. Neoplastic lymphocytes from a dog with Stage V lymphoma. Most of the lymphocytes are large and have fine chromatin, prominent nucleoli, and basophilic cytoplasm. A mitotic figure is present. Wright's stain, 1000X.

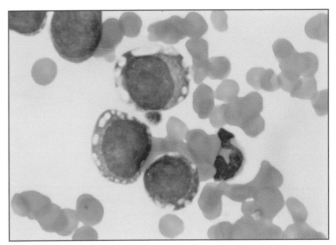

Figure 2. Neoplastic lymphocytes from a cat with lymphoma. The significance of the cytoplasmic vacuoles is unknown. Wright's stain, 1000X.

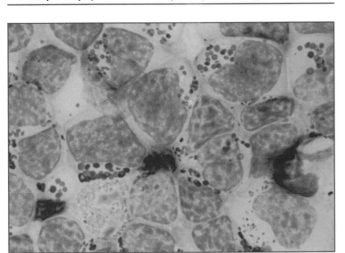

Figure 3. Neoplastic lymphocytes from a cat with alimentary lymphoma. The prominent azurophilic cytoplasmic granules are typical of granular lymphocytes. These cells likely are T lymphocytes or NK cells. Wright's stain, 1000X.

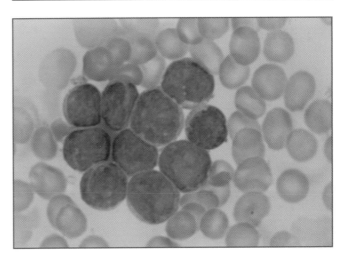

Figure 4. Neoplastic lymphocytes from a dog with Stage V lymphoma. The lymphocytes are small, the chromatin is clumped, nucleoli are inconspicuous, and there is minimal cytoplasm. It is sometimes difficult to differentiate between Stage V lymphoma involving a small cell type and chronic lymphoid leukemia. Wright's stain, 1000X.

circulating neoplastic lymphocytes, whereas dogs with acute lymphoid leukemia have only mild to moderate lymphadenomegaly and marked lymphocytosis. It also may be difficult to document that the neoplastic cells are lymphoid lineage, because immature lymphoid cells may resemble immature myeloid cells morphologically. Cell lineage is more specifically determined by cytochemical stains or immunophenotyping. Most lymphoid cells are negative for routine cytochemical staining reactions, whereas myeloid cells often are positive for several cytochemical stains (*Chapter 4, Table 1*). Immunophenotyping for lymphocyte

subsets may be useful as reagents become more readily available.

It is much more difficult to diagnose bone marrow infiltration in lymphoma if the cell type is a small or medium-sized lymphocyte (*Figure 4*). These cells more closely resemble the small lymphocytes that are present in healthy animals or the small to medium lymphocytes that are present in animals with lymphoid hyperplasia. In these cases, the diagnosis is supported by other clinical findings and by histologic evaluation of a bone marrow core biopsy.

Neoplastic proliferations are clonal disorders and inflammation is associated with polyclonal proliferations. The presence of one type of immunoglobulin light chain (kappa or lamda) or rearrangements of the T-cell receptor gene can be used to establish clonality of the proliferating lymphocytes. Lymphoma involving small lymphocytes is also difficult to distinguish from chronic lymphoid leukemia, which may be a clinical variation of the same disease.

Multiple Myeloma

Multiple myeloma is a neoplastic expansion of plasma cells that originates in the bone marrow and involves multiple sites. Multiple myeloma most often occurs in flat bones and osteolysis often occurs at the site of tumor involvement. Multiple myeloma typically is associated with abnormal production of one specific class of immunoglobulin, referred to as a paraprotein, monoclonal protein, or M component, which may be IgG or IgA.

Multiple myeloma is diagnosed by the presence of at least 2 of the following criteria: radiographic evidence of osteolytic lesions, a monoclonal gammopathy on serum protein electrophoresis, Bence Jones proteinuria, and plasma cell infiltration of bone marrow. Osteolytic lesions are recognized most commonly in vertebrae, long bones, and ribs. The monoclonal gammopathy is recognized as a narrow-based peak with a sharp apex on a serum protein electrophoretogram, most commonly in the beta or gamma region. Bence Jones proteins are light chain fragments of immunoglobulin that are sometimes produced in multiple myeloma. The light chain fragments are filtered by the glomeruli and can be detected by urine protein electrophoresis. Plasma cell infiltration of the bone marrow can be determined by a bone marrow aspirate. Other hematopoietic tissues like spleen and lymph node also may be infiltrated with neoplastic plasma cells.

Multiple myeloma has been reported in dogs and less commonly in cats. Clinical signs are variable and are related to neoplastic cell proliferation and/or abnormal immunoglobulin production. Skeletal lesions may be manifested as lameness, bone pain, and pathologic fractures. Neurologic signs may be associated with compressive lesions of the spinal cord from vertebral body tumor extension or hyperviscosity. Animals with hemorrhagic diatheses may present with epistaxsis, gingival bleeding, bruising, intermittent GI bleeding, ecchymosis, or petechiation.

Renal function abnormalities may occur from persistent hypercalcemia, hyperviscosity, or infiltration of the kidney parenchyma.

Laboratory abnormalities are variable. If anemia is present, it may be regenerative or non-regenerative. There may be leukocytosis or leukopenia. Normal platelet counts may be associated with abnormal platelet function, which may contribute to abnormal hemostasis. In some animals, pancytopenia is present. Rarely, neoplastic plasma cells are detected on peripheral blood films. Classically, there is an increased serum protein concentration with decreased albumin and increased globulin concentrations. In some cases, serum protein and globulin concentrations are normal. The abnormal immunoglobulin is recognized as a monoclonal pattern on a serum protein electrophoretogram. Decreased levels of normal immunoglobulins frequently occur and may be associated with an increased incidence of infection. The class of abnormal immunoglobulin can be determined by immunoelectrophoresis or isoelectric focusing, but this may not affect prognosis or treatment.

Bone marrow aspirates are recommended for animals with a provisional diagnosis of multiple myeloma. Aspiration of a lytic lesion is ideal but in some cases, bone marrow involvement is diffuse and aspiration of what appears to be unaffected bone will yield a diagnostic sample. In healthy animals, plasma cells are less than 2% of the nucleated cells in the bone marrow. Plasma cell numbers often are markedly increased in multiple myeloma. However, increased numbers of non-neoplastic plasma cells can occur with inflammation, and the distinction between multiple myeloma and plasma cell hyperplasia often cannot be made based only on numbers of plasma cells. Focal aggregates and dense sheets of plasma cells are more common in multiple myeloma than in plasma cell hyperplasia.

It is difficult to distinguish hyperplastic from neoplastic plasma cells based on morphology. Neoplastic plasma cells may appear well-differentiated, in which case they are recognized as large, round to oval cells with abundant, intensely basophilic cytoplasm and round, often eccentric nuclei with condensed chromatin (*Figure 5*). There may be a perinuclear clear zone, which represents the Golgi region. In some cases, plasma cells appear to have a ruffled, eosinophilic border (flame cells, *Figure 6*). Clear, crystalline, round to very irregularly shaped cytoplasmic inclusions called Russell bodies can sometimes be present. These

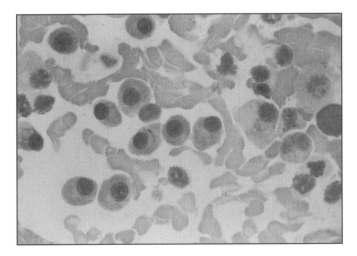

Figure 5. Plasma cells from a dog with multiple myeloma. This figure nicely illustrates the abundant basophilic cytoplasm, perinuclear clear zone, and eccentric nuclei characteristic of plasma cells. Wright's stain, 400X.

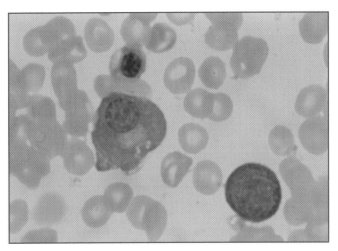

Figure 6. A plasma cell with a ruffled eosinophilic border. This type of plasma cell is called a flame cell. Wright's stain, 1000X.

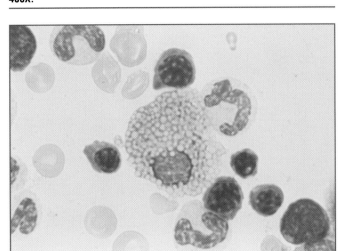

Figure 7. Mott cell illustrating the round, clear inclusions that likely are rough endoplasmic reticulum distended with antibody. Wright's stain, 1000X.

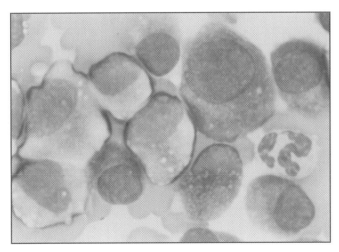

Figure 8. Anaplastic plasma cells from a lytic lesion of a dog with multiple myeloma. There is marked variation in cell size, nuclear size, and nuclear to cytoplasmic ratio. The basophilic cytoplasm, eccentric nuclei, and perinuclear clear zones present in some cells suggest that these cells are plasma cells. This dog had a monoclonal gammopathy and multiple lytic lesions. Wright's stain, 1000X.

may represent endoplasmic reticulum distended with antibody. Plasma cells with Russell bodies are called Mott cells (*Figure 7*).

Less differentiated plasma cells are even larger cells with large nuclei. The cytoplasm may be less basophilic, chromatin is less condensed, and nucleoli may be present. There may be marked variation in cell size, nuclear size, and nuclear to cytoplasmic ratio (*Figure 8*). These morphologic variations are typical of anaplastic plasma cells in some patients with multiple myeloma, but also can occur in marked plasma cell hyperplasia. In some cases, the plasma cells may be so anaplastic that recognition of cell lineage is

difficult. Ultrastructure and immunophenotypic determination of surface immunoglobulin may be used to identify the cells as plasma cells.

Monoclonal increases in IgM associated with neoplastic expansions of plasma cells are referred to as Waldenström's macroglobulinemia. This disease differs from multiple myeloma in that no bone lesions are present. The incidence of hyperviscosity syndrome is higher for plasma cells producing IgM than for IgA or IgG.

Monoclonal immunoglobulin production occasionally

occurs with chronic inflammation, usually in association with an infectious agent. Classic examples include dogs with chronic *Ehrlichia canis* infection and cats with feline infectious peritonitis virus infection. The overlap of clinical findings and laboratory abnormalities in animals with multiple myeloma and chronic inflammation often makes definitive diagnosis difficult. Recent development of more sensitive and specific assays for some of the infectious diseases that have been associated with monoclonal gammopathies likely will be useful in making the distinction between neoplastic and hyperplastic proliferations of plasma cells.

Plasma Cell Tumors

Plasma cell tumors (plasmacytomas) are solitary masses involving the gastrointestinal tract, respiratory tract, skin, or hematopoietic tissues other than the bone marrow. Secretory plasma cell tumors may be associated with monoclonal gammopathies. No osteolytic lesions are present because the bone marrow is not involved.

Leukemia

Neoplastic proliferation of hematopoietic cells that originates within the bone marrow is called leukemia. The presence of neoplastic cells in the blood is variable, even with marked bone marrow infiltration. Typically, there is marked leukocytosis due to large numbers of circulating neoplastic cells. A bone marrow aspirate is done to confirm the diagnosis of leukemia and classify the neoplastic cells. However, in occasional cases, so few circulating neoplastic cells are present that they are missed in routine blood film evaluation. Careful review of blood films often reveals the presence of a few neoplastic cells and a bone marrow aspirate is done to establish a diagnosis of leukemia.

Leukemias often are classified as acute or chronic, based on clinicopathologic findings, and lymphoid or myeloid, based on cell lineage. Determination of cell lineage for leukemic cells in dogs and cats is based on morphologic and cytochemical characteristics patterned after classification schemes used for leukemias in human beings. Morphologic and cytochemical evaluation of leukemic cells is performed on well-prepared peripheral blood and bone marrow aspirate smears by experienced veterinary clinical pathologists. High quality smears are essential for optimal evaluation. Immunophenotyping, cytogenetic analysis, and a variety of molecular techniques also are used to classify

leukemic cells in human beings. These gradually are being added as additional classification criteria for leukemic cells in dogs and cats. In human beings, classification of leukemias is very important in establishing a prognosis and designing specific treatment protocols. Ideally, similar progress will be made for classification of leukemias in dogs and cats so that rational decisions can be made about therapy.

Acute Lymphoblastic Leukemia

Acute lymphoblastic leukemia (ALL) involves infiltration of the bone marrow by immature, poorly differentiated lymphoid cells and is characterized by acute onset, aggressive behavior, and poor response to therapy. Clinical findings are nonspecific and include lethargy, anorexia, fever, pallor, vomiting, diarrhea, dyspnea, and bleeding diatheses. Abnormalities on physical exam are variable and include mild to moderate lymphadenomegaly, hepatosplenomegaly, joint swelling, bone pain, purpura, pleural effusion, various neuropathies, retinal hemorrhages or infiltrates, and chemosis.

Lymphocyte counts in ALL may range from 5,000/µl to greater than 100,000/µl. Most often there is marked lymphocytosis involving morphologically immature lymphoid cells. Severe non-regenerative anemia, neutropenia, and thrombocytopenia are common due to suppression of erythroid, myeloid and megakaryocytic proliferation. Lymph nodes, liver, spleen, bone, nervous tissue, and the GI tract also may be infiltrated with neoplastic lymphoid cells. Lymphadenomegaly, if present, usually is less dramatic than in lymphoma, and this may be useful in distinguishing ALL from lymphoma with bone marrow involvement.

The neoplastic lymphoid cells in ALL characteristically are large, round cells with a relatively high nuclear to cytoplasmic ratio, finely stippled to irregularly clumped chromatin, and one to several nucleoli (*Figure 9*). The cytoplasm may be moderately to markedly basophilic. Cytoplasmic vacuoles may be present but the significance of these is not known. In some cases, azurophilic cytoplasmic granules may be present, which suggests that the cells are a subset of T lymphocytes or NK cells called granular lymphocytes (*Figure 10*). The clinical relevance of this cell type in ALL in dogs and cats has not been determined. Lymphoid cells usually are negative for routine cytochemical staining reactions. ALL in cats most commonly involves T lymphocytes. Immunophenotyping has not been done in most cases of ALL in dogs. The bone marrow often appears hypercellular

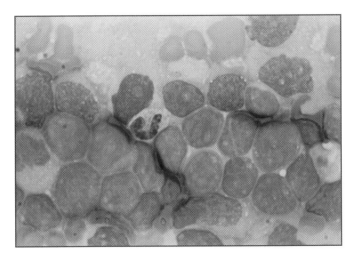

Figure 9. Neoplastic lymphoid cells from a dog with acute lymphoblastic leukemia. These cells are large and have finely stippled chromatin, prominent nucleoli, and basophilic cytoplasm. The bone marrow was markedly infiltrated with neoplastic lymphocytes. Wright's stain, 1000X.

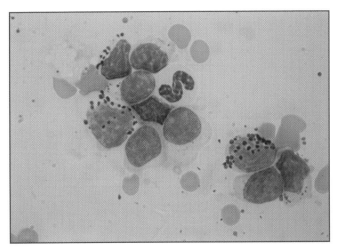

Figure 10. Neoplastic lymphocytes from a cat with granular lymphocyte leukemia. The azurophilic cytoplasmic granules are a unique morphologic feature of this subset of lymphocytes, which likely are T lymphocytes or NK cells. Wright's stain, 1000X.

due to marked infiltration with neoplastic lymphocytes. Usually, greater than 30% of the nucleated cells are neoplastic lymphocytes. Myeloid, erythroid, and megakaryocytic precursors usually are markedly decreased or absent.

Chronic Lymphocytic Leukemia

Chronic lymphocytic leukemia (CLL) appears to be relatively uncommon in dogs and cats but may go unrecognized because many animals with CLL appear clinically normal. The presence of leukemia often is discovered incidentally during routine hematologic screening. CLL is characterized by excessive numbers of circulating small lymphocytes, which morphologically appear well-differentiated. The majority of the neoplastic lymphocytes usually have condensed chromatin, inconspicuous nucleoli, and a small amount of cytoplasm. In some cases, up to 20% of the neoplastic lymphocytes appear immature. The neoplastic cells almost always are of B-cell origin in human beings. In contrast, CLL in dogs may be more commonly of T-cell origin with a CD4-, CD8+ phenotype.

If present, clinical signs are relatively nonspecific and include lethargy, anorexia, fever, vomiting, diarrhea, polyuria/polydipsia, and intermittent lameness. Physical findings may include mild to moderate peripheral lymphadenomegaly and hepatosplenomegaly. Skin involvement has been described in dogs.

The white blood cell (WBC) count typically is moderately to markedly increased due to lymphocytosis. Lymphocyte counts may range from 5,000/µl to more than

100,000/µl. CLL may be accompanied by mild to moderate non-regenerative anemia and normal or decreased numbers of platelets. Most dogs with CLL have normal serum globulin concentrations. However, hypogammaglobulinemia or hypergammaglobulinemia can occur. Monoclonal gammopathies have been reported in more than 50% of dogs with CLL, even when serum globulin concentrations are normal. The bone marrow is infiltrated with neoplastic lymphocytes. Infiltration of other hematopoietic tissues is variable.

It may be difficult to recognize bone marrow infiltration in CLL because the lymphocytes appear small and well differentiated (*Figure 11*). In healthy dogs and cats, less than 10% and 15% of all nucleated cells are small

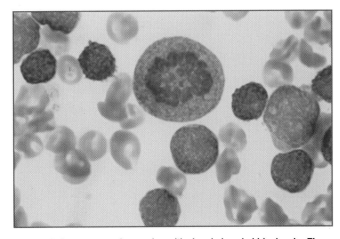

Figure 11. Bone marrow from a dog with chronic lymphoid leukemia. The lymphocytes are small and have condensed chromatin and inconspicuous nucleoli. A mitotic figure is present in the upper center. Wright's stain, 1000X.

lymphocytes, respectively. In CLL, usually greater than 20% of the nucleated cells are lymphocytes. It also may be difficult to distinguish CLL in the bone marrow from lymphoid hyperplasia or lymphoma involving a small cell type. In lymphoid hyperplasia, there may be increased numbers of plasma cells. In lymphoma, there usually is moderate to marked lymphadenomegaly and less dramatic lymphocytosis.

The clinical course is variable. Most commonly, the disease is progressive over several months or years, with eventual death due to infection, immune-mediated disorders, or debilitation. Blast crises rarely have been identified, but likely indicate a terminal event. Chemotherapy protocols have been described but treatment is controversial, since therapy may not prolong survival or improve quality of life.

Acute Myeloid Leukemia (AML)

- ❑ Undifferentiated or blast cell leukemia (AUL)
- ❑ Acute myeloblastic leukemia without maturation (M1)
- ❑ Acute myeloblastic leukemia with maturation (M2)
- ❑ Promyelocytic leukemia (M3)
- ❑ Myelomonocytic leukemia (M4)
- ❑ Monocytic leukemia (M5)
- ❑ Erythroleukemia (M6, M6-Er)
- ❑ Acute megakaryoblastic leukemia (M7)
- ❑ Myelodysplastic syndrome (MDS, MDS-Er)

Acute Myeloid Leukemia

The French-American-British Study Group classification system for acute myeloid leukemia (AML) used in human beings recently has been modified for dogs and cats and is outlined in *Figure 12*. For each determination, at least 200 nucleated cells are counted. First (Step 1), the percentage of all nucleated cells (ANC) that are erythroid cells is determined. Rubriblasts, prorubricytes, rubricytes, and metarubricytes are included as erythroid cells. ANC includes granulocytic, erythroid, and megakaryocytic precursors and differentiated cells. Lymphocytes, macrophages, mast cells, and plasma cells are excluded when calculating ANC.

Step 2 involves determination of the percentage of ANC that are blast cells. If less than 50% of ANC are erythroid cells from Step 1, then the percentage of ANC that are blast cells is determined from the sum of myeloblasts, monoblasts, and megakaryoblasts. Rubriblasts are excluded from this determination. If the sum of myeloblasts, monoblasts, and megakaryoblasts is greater than 30%, then the diagnosis is AML (M1-M5 or M7) or acute undifferentiated leukemia (AUL). AML is further classified based on cell morphology and cytochemical staining reactions. If less than 50% of ANC are erythroid cells (Step 1) and blast cells are less than 30% of ANC (Step 2), then the diagnosis is chronic myeloid leukemia (CML) or myelodysplastic syndrome (MDS). CML is distinguished from MDS based on the presence of marked leukocytosis in the peripheral blood and the absence of marked dysplastic changes in the bone marrow.

Step 3 is performed when erythroid cells in the bone marrow are greater than 50% of all nucleated cells (Step 1). Blast cell counts are first determined as a percentage of nonerythroid cells (NEC). In this determination, blast cells include myeloblasts, monoblasts, and megakaryoblasts, but not rubriblasts. If at this step, blast cells are greater than 30%, the diagnosis is erythroleukemia (M6). If blast cells (excluding rubriblasts) are less than 30% of ANC, then the diagnosis is MDS-Er. This is one of two ways to reach a diagnosis of MDS-Er.

Step 4 is similar to step 3 in that it is performed when erythroid cells are greater than 50% of ANC. In this step, however, blast cells include myeloblasts, monoblasts, megakaryoblasts, *and* rubriblasts. If erythroid cells are greater than 50% and all blasts, including rubriblasts, are equal to or greater than 30% of ANC, the diagnosis is a subtype of erythroleukemia called erythroleukemia with erythroid predominance (M6-Er). This condition previously was called erythremic myelosis. When erythroid cells are greater than 50% and all blasts, including rubriblasts, are less than 30% of ANC, the diagnosis is MDS-Er. This is the second way to reach a diagnosis of MDS-Er.

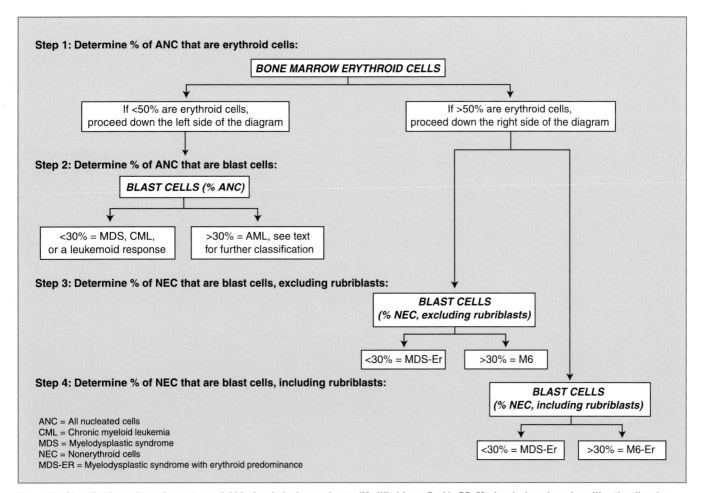

Step 1: Determine % of ANC that are erythroid cells:

BONE MARROW ERYTHROID CELLS

If <50% are erythroid cells, proceed down the left side of the diagram

If >50% are erythroid cells, proceed down the right side of the diagram

Step 2: Determine % of ANC that are blast cells:

BLAST CELLS (% ANC)

<30% = MDS, CML, or a leukemoid response

>30% = AML, see text for further classification

Step 3: Determine % of NEC that are blast cells, excluding rubriblasts:

BLAST CELLS
(% NEC, excluding rubriblasts)

<30% = MDS-Er

>30% = M6

Step 4: Determine % of NEC that are blast cells, including rubriblasts:

ANC = All nucleated cells
CML = Chronic myeloid leukemia
MDS = Myelodysplastic syndrome
NEC = Nonerythroid cells
MDS-ER = Myelodysplastic syndrome with erythroid predominance

BLAST CELLS
(% NEC, including rubriblasts)

<30% = MDS-Er

>30% = M6-Er

Figure 12. Classification scheme for acute myeloid leukemia in dogs and cats. (Modified from: Raskin RE. Myelopoiesis and myeloproliferative disorders. *Vet Clin North Am Small Anim Prac.* September, 1996; 1030.)

Subclassification of AML into 8 categories (AUL, M1, M2, M3, M4, M5, M6, and M7) is determined by the number and types of various blast cells present, which is based on morphologic characteristics in Romanowsky-stained blood and bone marrow smears and on cytochemical staining results. The most frequently used cytochemical reactions include myeloperoxidase (PO), naphthyl AS-D chloracetate esterase (CAE or specific esterase), alkaline phosphatase (ALP), and alpha-naphthyl butyrate (ANBE, nonspecific esterase). Chromosomal analysis and characterization of leukocyte specific membrane antigens by monoclonal antibodies are additional criteria used to classify leukemias in human beings. Electron microscopy and ultrastructural cytochemistry may be helpful. The clinical relevance of classification of AML in dogs and cats remains to be determined.

The diagnosis of acute myeloid leukemia in cats may be more difficult than in dogs. Recovery from marked leukopenia in cats (eg, after panleukopenia virus infection) may be associated with transient bone marrow findings that are similar to those described for cats with leukemia. The bone marrow may be hypercellular and there may be many immature granulocytes, some with giant, bizarre nuclear shapes. Repeat aspirates 1 or 2 weeks after the initial aspirate usually yield more normal cellularity and cellular morphology in cats with non-neoplastic disease, compared to cats with AML. AML in most cats is associated with FeLV infection.

Undifferentiated or Blast Cell Leukemia (AUL)

Undifferentiated leukemia has been used to describe acute myeloproliferative disorders in which the blast cells show no differentiation and the neoplastic cells are negative in cytochemical staining reactions. Typically, there is non-regenerative anemia accompanied by circulating neoplastic cells. Neutrophil and platelet counts are variable but often are decreased. The bone marrow is characterized by marked infiltration with large cells that have round to irregularly shaped nuclei, fine chromatin, prominent nucleoli, and basophilic, agranular cytoplasm. Undifferentiated leukemias may represent neoplastic transformation of an uncommitted stem cell. A characteristic primitive cell with a round, eccentric nucleus and a single, large cytoplasmic pseudopod has been described in cats with undifferentiated leukemia. In the past, these cells were called reticuloendothelial cells and the leukemia was called reticuloendotheliosis.

Acute Myeloblastic Leukemia without Maturation (M1)

AML without maturation (M1) is a disease of multipotential hematopoietic myeloid progenitor cells with a predominance of type I myeloblasts in the bone marrow. Type II myeloblasts (myeloblasts with a few small granules) are rare. Both types of blasts account for more than 90% of ANC. Differentiated granulocytes are less than 10% of non-erythroid cells (NEC) and may include segmented neutrophils, eosinophils, and monocytes. The number of myeloblasts in peripheral blood is variable. There may be leukopenia with only occasional myeloblasts or a striking leukocytosis with 100% myeloblasts. Morphologic differentiation of myeloblasts from lymphoblasts may be difficult. Myeloblasts are characterized by more finely dispersed chromatin, a more prominent nucleolus, and, in some cases, azurophilic cytoplasmic granules. There may be some maturation to promyelocytes through segmented neutrophils. The Auer rods characteristic of AML in humans have not been clearly identified in dogs and cats. In many cases, myeloblasts appear totally undifferentiated and cell lineage is determined by cytochemical reactions or ultrastructural features. More than 3% of the blasts should react positively for PO or CAE.

Acute Myeloblastic Leukemia with Maturation (M2)

Myeloblasts comprise more than 30% but less than 90% of ANC, with a variable proportion of type II myeloblasts. The M2 form of AML is characterized by maturation of myeloblasts to neutrophilic promyelocytes and later stages of development, which account for more than 10% of NEC, with a predominance or disproportionate number of progranulocytes (*Figure 13*). Eosinophils and basophils may be

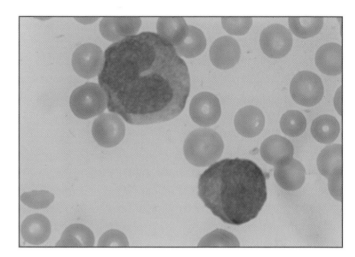

Figure 13. Immature myeloid cells from a dog with acute myeloid leukemia (M2). Wright's stain, 1000X.

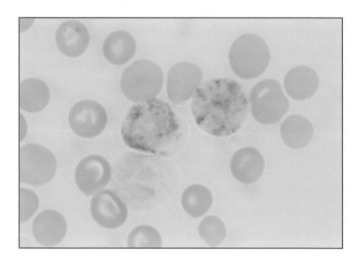

Figure 14. Two myeloid precursors from a dog with acute myeloid leukemia (M2). The reddish granules indicate positive staining for CAE, which is characteristic for cells of the neutrophil series. CAE stain, 1000X.

present, but if either predominate, the terms eosinophilic and basophilic leukemia have been used. Monocytes are less than 20% of NEC. Differentiated cells may appear hypogranular and have poorly lobated nuclei. Atypical myeloblasts with bilobed or reniform nuclei may resemble monocytes. Cytochemical staining for PO and CAE can be used to confirm the diagnosis (*Figure 14*).

Promyelocytic Leukemia (M3)

Promyelocytic AML (M3) has not been reported in dogs and cats. Hypergranular myeloblasts and promyelocytes, which are intensely myeloperoxidase positive, comprise the majority of cells in this form of AML in human beings.

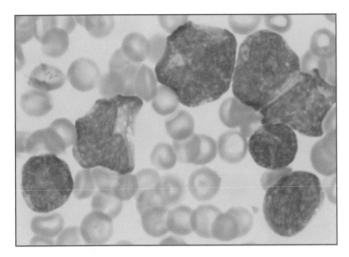

Figure 15. Neoplastic monocytes from a dog with acute monocytic leukemia (M5b). Immature monocytes are characterized by nuclei with irregular or clefted outlines. Wright's stain, 1000X.

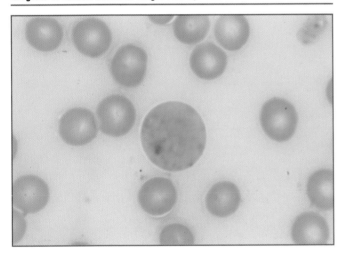

Figure 16. Neoplastic monocyte from a dog with acute myeloid leukemia (M5b). The diffuse reddish-brown staining indicates a positive reaction for ANBE activity, which is characteristic for monocytic cells. ANBE stain, 1000X.

Myelomonocytic Leukemia (M4)

Myelomonocytic leukemia (AMMOL; M4) is characterized by both neutrophilic and monocytic differentiation. Myeloblasts and monoblasts together are more than 30% of ANC. Differentiated granulocytes and monocytes each are more than 20% of NEC. Monocytic cells typically have pleomorphic nuclei and cytoplasmic vacuoles. Definitive diagnosis depends upon cytochemical stains to demonstrate nonspecific esterase activity in monocytic cells and specific esterase activity in neutrophilic cells. Spontaneous AMMOL appears to be one of the more common myeloproliferative diseases in dogs and cats.

Monocytic Leukemia (M5)

Monocytic leukemia (M5) is uncommon in dogs and cats. White blood cell counts are variable but usually there is monocytosis with many immature cells. Immature monocytic cells are characterized by nuclei with finely stippled to reticular chromatin, an irregular or clefted outline, and nuclear membrane foldings (*Figure 15*). There are 2 subtypes of monocytic leukemia. In poorly-differentiated monoblastic leukemia (M5a), the proliferating cells are primarily monoblasts with minimal differentiation to promonocytes or monocytes. Monoblasts and promonocytes constitute more than 80% of ANC. In the differentiated form of monocytic leukemia (M5b), more than 30% but less than 80% of the ANC are monoblasts, and there is prominent maturation to mature monocytes. Less than 20% of ANC are granulocytic cells in M5a and M5b. The majority of cells in M5a and M5b react positively with nonspecific esterase staining (*Figure 16*).

Erythroleukemia (M6, M6-Er)

AML is classified as M6 when more than 50% of ANC are erythroid precursor cells and more than 30% of the cells are myeloblasts, monoblasts, and megakaryoblasts. In this case, the blast cell count excludes rubriblasts. AML is classified as M6 with erythroid predominance (M6-Er) when the erythroid component is more than 50% of ANC and a blast cell count that includes rubriblasts is more than 30% of ANC. The term erythremic myelosis previously was used for cats with M6-Er. The CBC typically is characterized by high numbers of immature erythroid cells (metarubricytes, rubricytes, and in some cases, prorubricytes and rubriblasts), in the presence of marked nonregenerative anemia. Morphologic abnormalities in erythroid precursors are common and include multinucleation, multilobulated nuclei, nuclear fragments, giant forms and megaloblastic changes (*Figure 17*). Abnormal megakaryocytes may be present. M6 frequently progresses to other forms of acute myeloid leukemia (M1, M2, or M4). M6 and M6-Er occur in cats but are rare in dogs.

Acute Megakaryoblastic Leukemia (M7)

Acute megakaryoblastic leukemia (M7) is rare in dogs and cats and is characterized by circulating micromegakaryocytes and undifferentiated megakaryoblasts. Platelet counts are variable and may be markedly

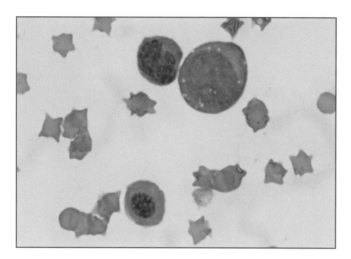

Figure 17. Neoplastic cells from a cat with erythroleukemia. The cell in the lower left is a megaloblastic erythroid cell and the cell in the upper right resembles an erythroid precursor. Wright's stain, 1000X.

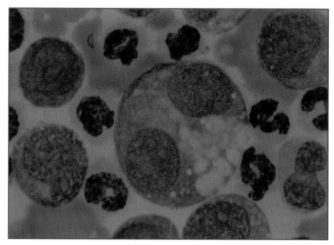

Figure 19. Neoplastic megakaryocytic cell from a dog with megakaryoblastic leukemia. There were frequent binucleate and multinucleate cells and numerous cells had cytoplasmic vacuoles. (Bone marrow smear courtesy of Dr. Joanne Messick.)

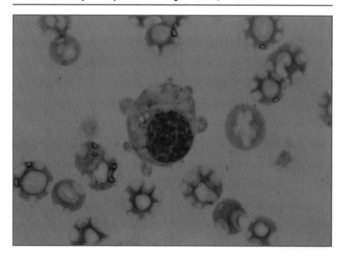

Figure 18. Abnormal platelet with retained nuclear material from a dog with megakaryoblastic leukemia. Wright's stain, 1000X. (Blood film courtesy of Dr. Joanne Messick.)

decreased. Morphologically abnormal platelets may be present (*Figure 18*). Hemorrhagic diatheses have been reported, presumably due to abnormal platelet function. More than 30% of bone marrow ANC are megakaryoblasts in M7. Megakaryoblasts are difficult to identify morphologically by light microscopy. Frequent binucleate or multinucleate cells with conspicuous cytoplasmic blebs, vacuolation, and variable granulation have been described (*Figure 19*).

Cytochemical staining and ultrastructural morphology can be used to aid in identification of megakaryoblasts. Megakaryoblasts stain positively for acetylcholinesterase and periodic acid-Schiff. The leukemic cells are negative

for routine peroxidase activity but are positive for platelet peroxidase activity at the ultrastructural level. Megakaryo-blasts are characterized ultrastructurally by cytoplasmic demarcation membrane systems, an extensive open canalicular system, numerous filopodia, and alpha granules. Immunophenotyping for platelet glycoproteins Ib, IIb/IIIa, IIIa, or factor VIII-related antigen (von Willebrand's factor) also may be helpful to identify megakaryoblasts.

Myelodysplastic Syndrome (MDS, MDS-Er)

Myelodysplastic syndromes (MDS and MDS-Er) have been sub-classified in human medicine based on the predominant cell type and biologic behavior. Similar subclassification has been proposed for MDS in dogs and cats but only MDS and MDS-Er will be discussed here. MDS and MDS-Er are rare in dogs and cats and are characterized by hypercellular or normocellular bone marrow with peripheral cytopenias. Rarely, the bone marrow is hypocellular. MDS and MDS-Er in cats are associated with FeLV infection whereas the etiology in dogs is unknown. MDS is diagnosed when the erythroid component is less than 50% and fewer than 30% of ANC are blast cells. The diagnosis is MDS-Er when the erythroid component is greater than 50% and either myeloblasts and monoblasts combined are less than 30% of the NEC or ANC, or when myeloblasts, monoblasts, and rubriblasts are less than 30% of NEC.

Dysplastic changes frequently are present and include:

dyserythropoiesis, characterized by binucleate cells, nuclear fragmentation, and megaloblastosis; dysgranulopoiesis, characterized by giant metamyelocytes and band neutrophils, hypogranularity, nuclear hyposegmentation, and pseudo Pelger-Huët nuclei; and dysthrombopoiesis, characterized by micromegakaryocytes with dispersed or fragmented nuclei and increased numbers of cells with unilobed or bilobed nuclei.

MDS is characterized by anemia, thrombocytopenia, and neutropenia, occurring singly or in various combinations. Clinical findings are related to the cytopenias and include lethargy, weakness, infections and bleeding. Hepatomegaly and/or splenomegaly may be present. The clinical course is variable. In human beings, progression to overt leukemia is more likely if there are qualitative or quantitative abnormalities of more than one cell line, the peripheral cytopenias are severe, chromosomal changes are present, or there are abnormalities of *in vitro* cell growth. Progression of MDS to AML has been described in dogs and cats but specific abnormalities associated progression have not been identified.

Chronic Myeloproliferative Disorders

- Chronic myeloid leukemia (CML)
- Polycythemia vera/
  Primary polycythemia (PV)
- Essential thrombocythemia (ET)

Chronic Myeloproliferative Disorders

Myeloproliferative disorders can be classified based on the degree of differentiation of the primary cell line involved. Chronic myeloproliferative diseases are characterized by excessive proliferation of terminally differentiated blood cells and include chronic myelogenous leukemia (CML), polycythemia vera (PV), and essential thrombocythemia (ET). Clinical findings are relatively nonspecific. Diagnosis of chronic myeloproliferative disorders is based on characteristic abnormalities in peripheral blood and bone marrow that are specific for each disease. In general, chronic myeloproliferative diseases are less aggressive and have a better prognosis than acute myeloproliferative diseases.

Chronic Myeloid Leukemia

Chronic myelogenous leukemia (CML) is uncommon in dogs and has not been clearly documented in cats. Many reports of myelogenous leukemia in dogs and cats have failed to distinguish CML from AML. Diagnosis of CML is difficult and is based on the presence of persistent marked leukocytosis with a predominance of mature neutrophils, a slowly progressive clinical course, and absence of inflammatory disease or other malignant neoplasms. CML in human beings results from neoplastic transformation of a pluripotent stem cell. Although multiple cell lineages are involved, clinical features usually are limited to excessive numbers of granulocytes, likely related to increased production, prolonged accumulation, or both. Presumably, a similar stem cell transformation occurs in CML in dogs and cats.

Clinical signs associated with CML are nonspecific and include lethargy, inappetence, and weakness. Hepatomegaly and splenomegaly may be present. White blood cell counts in CML usually are greater than 100,000/µl. All stages of development of the neutrophil series are present with a progressive increase in the percentages of more mature cells. The majority of cells are segmented neutrophils. Myeloblasts usually do not exceed 3% of the nucleated cells in peripheral blood or bone marrow, and do not exceed 30% of ANC in the bone marrow. The eosinophilia and basophilia associated with CML in humans is not a consistent finding in dogs with CML. Moderate non-regenerative anemia is common in dogs with CML.

Infections, immune-mediated diseases, and other malignant neoplasms are more common causes of marked leukocytosis than CML. If the total leukocyte count exceeds 50,000/µl, the term leukemoid reaction is often used to indicate that the cause of the marked leukocytosis is non-neoplastic. Physical examination and other laboratory findings may be helpful in establishing a non-neoplastic cause for the leukocytosis. A biopsy of an enlarged liver or spleen may reveal neoplastic infiltrates in CML. In human beings, neutrophils from patients with CML have low alkaline phosphatase activity and a distinct chromosomal abnormality that distinguishes them from non-neoplastic neutrophils. These tests have not been useful in the diagnosis of CML in dogs.

CML may be classified under MDS because the blast cell counts are less than 30% of ANC and the erythroid component is less than 50% of the cells in the bone marrow. However, MDS is associated with peripheral blood cytopenias whereas CML is characterized by marked leukocytosis. The dysplastic changes present in the bone marrow in MDS usually are not present or are much more subtle in CML. A bone marrow aspirate will reveal a marked increase in the M:E due to a marked increase in myeloid precursors and erythroid hypoplasia. Often, myeloid maturation appears orderly and it is only by excluding other causes of myeloid hyperplasia that the diagnosis of CML can be made.

In human beings, the chronic phase of CML is unstable. At some point, the disease undergoes transformation to an aggressive leukemia, and the majority of cells in peripheral blood and bone marrow resemble blast cells ("blast crisis"). This phenomenon has been described in dogs with CML. Long-term prognosis for CML is guarded, even with therapy, because of the likelihood of disease progression.

Polycythemia Vera

Polycythemia vera (PV) or primary polycythemia is uncommon in dogs and rare in cats and is characterized by increased RBC mass in the presence of normal oxygen saturation and normal or low serum erythropoietin concentration. RBC count, hemoglobin concentration, and packed cell volume are increased. Packed cell volumes are in the range of 65% to 80%. PV in human beings is a stem cell disorder characterized by erythrocytosis, leukocytosis, and thrombocytosis. Leukocytosis is not as common in dogs or cats with PV and in dogs with PV, thrombocytopenia is more common than thrombocytosis. Clinical findings include erythema, polydipsia, polyuria, hemorrhage and neurologic signs, many of which may result from hyperviscosity. Splenomegaly occurs in 75% of humans and dogs with PV. In contrast to the bone marrow hyperplasia seen in human beings, bone marrow aspirates from dogs with PV usually appear normal and may not be helpful in the diagnosis. PV may progress to myelofibrosis or AML.

The diagnosis of PV depends upon eliminating other causes of polycythemia. Dehydration and splenic contraction cause *relative* polycythemia, but RBC mass is normal.

In contrast, *absolute* polycythemia is characterized by an actual increase in RBC mass. Absolute polycythemia may be primary (PV) or secondary. Secondary polycythemia is characterized by increased RBC mass as a result of increased serum erythropoietin in response to tissue hypoxia, as in right-to-left cardiovascular shunts or chronic pulmonary disease, or from autonomous production, as in certain renal diseases (renal cysts, hydronephrosis, polycystic kidney disease) or tumors that secrete erythropoietin (eg, renal carcinoma).

Essential Thrombocythemia

Essential thrombocythemia (ET) (primary or idiopathic thrombocythemia, primary thrombocytosis) is a clonal disorder of hematopoietic stem cells that primarily involves cells of the megakaryocytic series. ET recently has been described in dogs and cats and must be differentiated from other causes of increased platelet number. Physiologic and reactive thrombocytosis are transient and platelet counts rarely exceed 1,000,000/µl. Physiologic thrombocytosis occurs when platelets are released from splenic or extrasplenic storage pools. Reactive thrombocytosis occurs with iron deficiency, acute and chronic inflammatory disorders, hepatic cirrhosis, recovery from severe hemorrhage, hemolytic anemia, trauma, surgery, splenectomy, certain solid tumors, and collagen vascular diseases. Thrombocytosis also may be associated with any of the chronic myeloproliferative disorders.

Clinical findings may include anemia secondary to chronic blood loss and pseudohyperkalemia from marked thrombocytosis. The spleen may be enlarged due to extramedullary hematopoiesis or contracted due to splenic atrophy. As in other chronic myeloproliferative disorders, leukocytosis with eosinophilia and basophilia have been reported in humans and dogs with ET. Bleeding is more common than thrombosis and either may be associated with abnormal platelet function. Platelets may exhibit abnormal morphologic characteristics including giant-sized platelets, hypo- and hypergranularity, cytoplasmic vacuolation, and bizarre shapes. These are nonspecific changes typical of platelet dysplasia in other myeloproliferative disorders. In contrast to acute megakaryoblastic leukemia, megakaryoblasts and micromegakaryocytes are not found in peripheral blood, liver, or spleen in ET.

The bone marrow is hyperplastic with moderate hyper-proliferation of erythroid and myeloid cell lines. There is marked megakaryocytic hyperplasia in the bone marrow but megakaryoblasts are less than 30% of ANC. Megakaryocytes may exhibit abnormal morphology such as increased size, redundant cytoplasm, and increased nuclear lobation. Morphologic identification of megakaryocytes and megakaryoblasts may be confirmed as described above.

Miscellaneous Myeloproliferative Disorders

☐ Myelofibrosis
☐ Eosinophilic leukemia
☐ Basophilic leukemia
☐ Mast cell leukemia
☐ Malignant histiocytosis
☐ Metastatic neoplasia

Miscellaneous Myeloproliferative Disorders

Myelofibrosis

Myelofibrosis previously has been considered as one of the chronic myeloproliferative disorders but clonal prolifera-tions of fibroblasts have not been described. Myelofibrosis most appropriately is used as a histologic term to denote excess collagen in bone marrow. The fibrosis may result from megakaryocytic or platelet-derived growth factors that stimulate increases in fibroblast number and secretion of col-lagen. Both myeloproliferative and lymphoproliferative dis-orders may terminate in myelofibrosis and this disorder may be secondary to bone marrow damage. Myelofibrosis has been reported only rarely in dogs and cats and includes cases secondary to megakaryocytic leukemia, irradiation, bone marrow necrosis, hematopoietic neoplasia, pyruvate kinase deficiency, familial nonspherocytic hemolytic anemia, and FeLV infection. Myelofibrosis is characterized by bone mar-row fibrosis accompanied by poikilocytosis, anisocytosis, leukoerythroblastosis, and splenomegaly with extramedullary hematopoiesis. There may be anemia and thrombocytopenia. Megakaryocytes may appear morphologi-cally abnormal and megakaryocytopoiesis may be ineffective.

Fibrosis prevents adequate bone marrow aspiration and diagnosis of myelofibrosis depends on bone marrow biopsy.

Eosinophilic leukemia

In human beings, eosinophilic leukemia is considered a variant of AML in which a high proportion of cells has eosinophilic differentiation. Rarely, the disease is a variant of CML. Eosinophilic leukemia is difficult to differentiate from hypereosinophilic syndromes associated with skin and respiratory disorders, parasitism, and inflammatory bowel disease. Eosinophilic leukemia usually is characterized by a predominance of immature eosinophils in the peripheral blood, including segmented eosinophils and eosinophilic bands, metamyelocytes, myelocytes, and myeloblasts. However, more mature forms have predominated in some cats with eosinophilic leukemia. The eosinophilia associated with hypereosinophilic syndrome usually includes segment-ed, bilobed, banded, and occasional metamyelocyte forms. Eosinophilic leukemia is rare in cats and dogs. Cats with spontaneous eosinophilic leukemia usually are negative for FeLV infection, but the disease has been produced experi-mentally with FeLV. Bone marrow aspirates are character-ized by hypercellularity with a predominance of eosinophilic precursors. Immature stages of development predominate and there may be morphologic atypia of the neoplastic cells (*Figure 20*).

Basophilic leukemia

Basophilic leukemia as a variant of AML in human

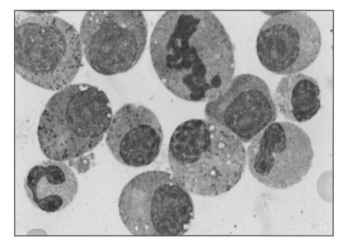

Figure 20. Bone marrow from a cat with eosinophilic leukemia. Numerous eosinophil precursors are present and there is very little differentiation to mature eosinophils. Wright's stain, 1000X. (Bone marrow smear courtesy of Dr. Cheryl Swenson.)

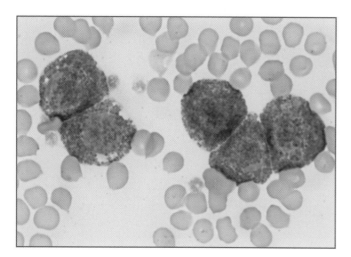

Figure 21. Neoplastic mast cells from a cat with mast cell leukemia. Mast cells are characterized by the presence of numerous purple cytoplasmic granules. Wright's stain, 1000X.

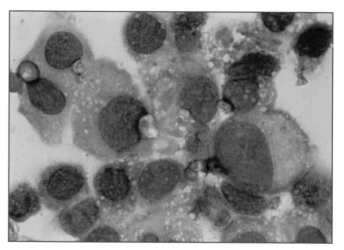

Figure 22. Neoplastic mast cells from a dog with systemic mastocytosis. These mast cells are very anaplastic based on marked variation in cell size, nuclear size, nuclear to cytoplasmic ratio, and minimal granularity. Wright's stain, 1000X.

beings is extremely rare. Most cases of basophilic leukemia in humans have a chronic course and evolve as a phase of CML. The disease is diagnosed by the presence of neoplastic basophils in peripheral blood and bone marrow. Neoplastic basophils may be difficult to differentiate from mast cells since neoplastic basophils may have hyposegmented nuclei and granule development may be aberrant. Cytochemical staining with omegaexonuclease may be useful in identifying poorly differentiated basophils. Basophilic leukemia is extremely rare in dogs and cats. Basophilic leukemia in cats is associated with FeLV infection whereas the etiology in dogs is unknown.

Mast cell leukemia

Mast cell leukemia and systemic mastocytosis often are used interchangeably in the veterinary literature and both terms imply a neoplastic proliferation of mast cells. However, mastocythemia also may occur in association with non-neoplastic disorders, such as intestinal or pulmonary inflammatory diseases. Mast cell leukemia in dogs is uncommon and usually is associated with systemic dissemination of primary cutaneous mast cell tumors. Mast cell leukemia in cats also is relatively uncommon. In cats, mast cell leukemia occurs from primary infiltration of hematopoietic organs with neoplastic mast cells. Unlike many hematopoietic disorders in cats, mast cell leukemia is unassociated with FeLV infection.

Clinical findings in mast cell leukemia include anorexia, vomiting, diarrhea, lymphadenopathy, splenomegaly, and hepatomegaly. Gastric ulcers have been described in dogs and cats with mast cell leukemia. Eosinophilia, basophilia, and coagulation abnormalities appear to be more common in dogs than in cats with mast cell leukemia. Circulating mast cells are variable in dogs with mast cell leukemia. Mast cells are round cells with round nuclei and cytoplasmic granules (*Figure 21*). Mast cell granules stain purple with Wright-Giemsa stain, but in some cases very few granules are present. The granules in mast cells may not stain with some commercial quick stains.

Bone marrow aspiration may be more sensitive than peripheral blood and buffy coat smears in detecting mast cell leukemia. Neoplastic mast cells often occur as dense aggregates or sheets within the bone marrow. The presence of more than 1% mast cells in bone marrow of adequate to increased cellularity is supportive of a diagnosis of mast cell leukemia, but increased numbers of mast cells have been reported in non-neoplastic diseases. Dogs with aplastic anemia may have 2% to 20% mast cells in the bone marrow, but the cellularity in these samples usually is low. Neoplastic mast cells may appear well-differentiated or anaplastic in dogs and cats with mast cell leukemia. Anaplastic mast cells are characterized by increased size, multinucleation, and poorly granulated cytoplasm (*Figure 22*). Occasional binucleate and multinucleate cells may be present. Erythrophagocytosis has been observed in a few cases of mast cell leukemia.

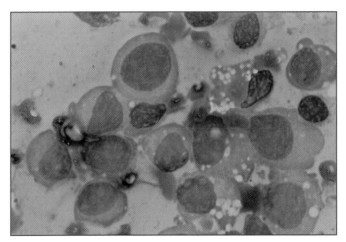

Figure 23. Malignant histiocytes from a dog with malignant histiocytosis. These cells are characterized by their large size and abundant cytoplasm. There is moderate to marked variation in cell size and nuclear size. Wright's stain, 1000X.

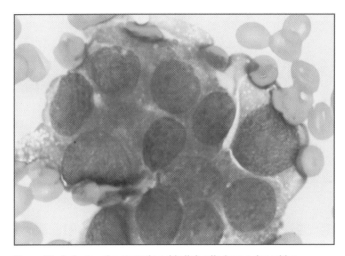

Figure 25. A cluster of metastatic epithelial cells from a dog with a mammary adenocarcinoma. The acinar formation shown in the cells in the upper left is typical of neoplastic glandular epithelial cells. Wright's stain, 1000X.

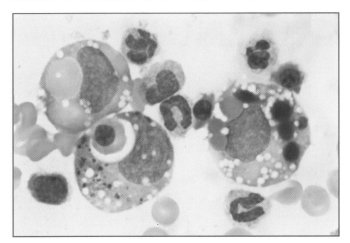

Figure 24. Malignant histiocytes from a dog with malignant histiocytosis. These cells have phagocytized erythroid precursors. Wright's stain, 1000X.

Malignant histiocytosis

Malignant histiocytosis (MH) is a systemic, neoplastic proliferation of macrophage-like cells called histiocytes. MH is uncommon in dogs and rare in cats. There is a breed predisposition for Bernese Mountain Dogs, Flat-coated Retrievers, Rottwiellers, and Golden Retrievers, and there appears to be a sex predilection for males. Clinical features associated with MH are nonspecific and include lethargy, anorexia, weight loss, and respiratory and neurologic abnormalities. There may be lymphadenomegaly, hepatosplenomegaly, and regenerative or non-regenerative anemia. The bone marrow often is infiltrated with anaplastic histiocytes. These cells are characterized by their large size, abundant cytoplasm, and bizarre nuclear shapes

(*Figure 23*). Nuclear chromatin is finely stippled or irregularly clumped and nucleoli may be prominent. There is marked anisocytosis and anisokaryosis. Binucleate and multinucleate cells often are present and there may be bizarre mitotic figures. Frequently, moderate numbers of cells with phagocytic activity are identified with erythroid and myeloid precursors in their cytoplasm (*Figure 24*). Definitive diagnosis of MH is made histologically but cell lineage is not always easily determined. Differentials include poorly differentiated carcinoma and non-neoplastic histiocytic proliferations. Malignant histiocytes are positive for ANBE, lysozyme, α-1 antitrypsin, and α-1 chymotrypsin.

Metastatic neoplasia

Common hematologic abnormalities in adult human beings with initial presentation of solid tumors in the bone marrow include anemia, leukocytosis, thrombocytopenia, and leukoerythroblastosis. A bone marrow may be performed in these patients to evaluate hematologic abnormalities and fever of unknown origin. Similar hematologic changes have been reported in a dog with metastatic pancreatic adenocarcinoma. Metastasis to the bone marrow occurs most commonly with hematopoietic tumors arising outside the marrow, such as mast cell tumors of the skin, and with carcinomas. Metastatic carcinoma is recognized by the presence of clumps or clusters of anaplastic cells (*Figure 25*). In some animals with myelophthisis associated with metastatic neoplasia, very few hematopoietic cells are present in the bone marrow.

CASE 1

SIGNALMENT: Five-year-old spayed female Cocker Spaniel dog
HISTORY: Acute onset of depression, lethargy, and petechiae on mucous membranes.

TP	(g/dl)	7.2
PCV	(%)	12
Hb	(g/dl)	3.5
RBC	(10^{12}/L)	1.50
MCV	(fl)	80
MCHC	(g/dl)	28
Reticulocytes	(10^9/L)	300
Platelets	(10^9/L)	15.0
WBC	(10^9/L)	55.5
nRBC	(10^9/L)	5.0
Seg. neutrophils	(10^9/L)	42.6
Band neutrophils	(10^9/L)	2.8
Lymphocytes	(10^9/L)	0.6
Monocytes	(10^9/L)	3.9
Eosinophils	(10^9/L)	0.6

HEMOGRAM DESCRIPTION:

Macrocytic, hypochromic anemia with thrombocytopenia. Spherocytes and macroplatelets are seen (*Figure 1*). There is a marked leukocytosis that is characterized by a neutrophilia with a left shift, monocytosis, and lymphopenia.

BONE MARROW EXAMINATION:

The sample is highly cellular, and the M:E ratio is 2.0. Megakaryocytes are markedly increased in number (*Figure 2*). Erythroid and myeloid cell lines are also increased in number. The maturation sequences of the erythroid and myeloid lines are orderly and go to completion. Occasional lymphocytes and plasma cells are seen. Hemosiderin is present.

Interpretation

Spherocytosis with a regenerative anemia in combination with a thrombocytopenia is compatible with immune-mediated hemolytic anemia (IHA) and thrombocytopenia (ITP). Generalized bone marrow hyperplasia and a peripheral leukocytosis usually accompany IHA and ITP. Hyperplasia of both erythroid and myeloid cell lines results in a normal M:E ratio. If a regenerative response is evident on the hemogram, it is usually unnecessary to perform a bone marrow evaluation. However, it may be helpful to determine if the bone marrow from a patient with ITP has increased numbers of megakaryocytes, compatible with productive response in this cell line. Rarely, antibodies may be directed at early erythroid or megakaryocytic precursors. This results in hypoplasia of those cells lines in the marrow, an appearance of maturation arrest, and a non-regenerative picture peripherally.

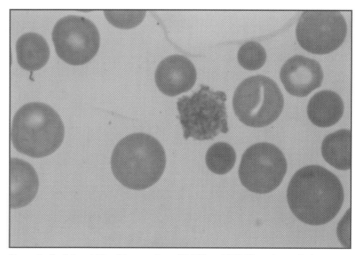

Figure 1. Peripheral blood from a dog with IHA and ITP. There is marked anisocytosis and polychromasia. Spherocytes are present. In the center is a macroplatelet. Wright's stain, 1000X.

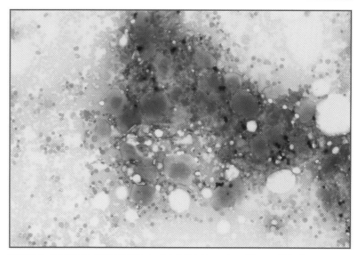

Figure 2. A particle of bone marrow from the same dog. The particle is very cellular and there is generalized hyperplasia of the marrow. Megakaryocytic hyperplasia is prominent. Hemosiderin may be seen as black staining material within the cluster of cells. Wright's stain, 1000X.

CASE 2

SIGNALMENT: Two-year-old female Chow Chow dog

HISTORY: Acute onset of bilateral epistaxis.

TP	(g/dl)	4.3
PCV	(%)	10
Hb	(g/dl)	3.3
RBC	(10^{12}/L)	1.67
MCV	(fl)	60
MCHC	(g/dl)	32.5
Reticulocytes	(10^9/L)	none
Platelets	(10^9/L)	22.0
WBC	(10^9/L)	1.7
Seg. neutrophils	(10^9/L)	0.9
Band neutrophils	(10^9/L)	0.1
Lymphocytes	(10^9/L)	0.6
Monocytes	(10^9/L)	0.1

HEMOGRAM DESCRIPTION:

Marked pancytopenia and a lack of a reticulocytosis despite a severe anemia.

BONE MARROW EXAMINATION:

The bone marrow is hypercellular and megakaryocytes are normal in number. The M:E ratio is 10.0 due to an apparent granulocytic hyperplasia and probable erythroid hypoplasia (*Figure 3*). The granulocytic cell line shows a left shift. This is compatible with either consumption and depletion of the maturation pool or early stages of recovery from the leukopenia. There is a marked increase in numbers of normal-appearing histiocytes. Many of the histiocytes are exhibiting cytophagia of erythrocytes, neutrophils and platelets (*Figure 4*).

Interpretation

A pancytopenia in conjunction with histiocytic hyperplasia in the bone marrow is compatible with hemophagocytic syndrome, which represents an overzealous, reactive response that develops secondary to inflammatory, metabolic, or neoplastic disease. Phagocytosis of blood elements by histiocytes may contribute to the cytopenias. Leukopenia with a left shift may develop secondary to consumption by an inflammatory process. Disseminated intravascular coagulation initiated by an inflammatory or neoplastic process also may contribute to the thrombocytopenia. Additional tests to evaluate the coagulation system, eg, measurement of fibrin degradation products (FDP), prothrombin time (PT), and activated partial thromboplastin time (APTT), may support this diagnosis. In addition to hemolysis, hemorrhage secondary to the thrombocytopenia likely contributed to both the anemia and low TP. Acute blood loss and hemolysis can present as a non-regenerative anemia if there was inadequate time between onset of anemia and evaluation of the CBC to allow for the bone marrow to respond. Anemia of chronic disease may be superimposed in these cases, producing a sluggish regenerative response. In this dog, all cell lines showed recovery after appropriate therapy was instituted.

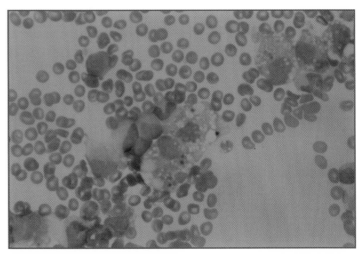

▲ Figure 3. Bone marrow from a dog with hemophagocytic syndrome. There are increased numbers of well-differentiated histiocytes. These macrophages appear actively phagocytic. Wright's stain, 400X.

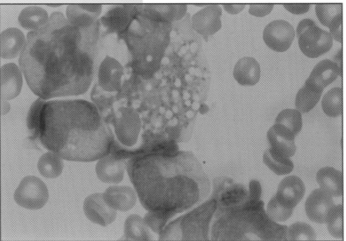

◀ Figure 4. Higher power view of Figure 3. Granulocytic myelocytes and a mitotic figure are seen. The histiocyte in the center of the field has phagocytized several RBCs and platelets. Wright's stain, 1000X.

CASE 3

SIGNALMENT: Twelve-year-old spayed female DSH cat

HISTORY: Gradual onset of depression, lethargy, and weight loss. Polyuric and polydipsic for 1 month.

TP	(g/dl)	8.5
PCV	(%)	12
Hb	(g/dl)	4.1
RBC	(10^{12}/L)	2.66
MCV	(fl)	45
MCHC	(g/dl)	34
Reticulocytes	(10^9/L)	none
Platelets	(10^9/L)	adequate
WBC	(10^9/L)	10.3
Seg. neutrophils	(10^9/L)	8.0
Band neutrophils	(10^9/L)	0.3
Lymphocytes	(10^9/L)	1.5
Monocytes	(10^9/L)	0.5

HEMOGRAM DESCRIPTION:

Severe normocytic, normochromic, non-regenerative anemia.

PERTINENT BIOCHEMISTRY DATA:

The cat is azotemic with elevated serum creatinine and serum urea nitrogen. Specific gravity from multiple urine samples ranged between 1.015 and 1.020.

BONE MARROW EXAMINATION:

The cellularity appears normal and the M:E ratio is 10.2. Megakaryocytes are adequate in number. Myeloid precursors appear adequate in number and the maturation sequence is orderly and goes to completion. There are decreased numbers of erythroid precursors, but cellular morphology appears normal (*Figure 5*).

Interpretation

Azotemia and the inability to concentrate the urine in the presence of dehydration (elevated TP) is compatible with renal disease. Renal failure is often associated with a severe non-regenerative anemia due to lack of adequate erythropoietin production by the kidney. Myeloid and megakaryocytic production may be maintained while erythroid production is markedly suppressed. Erythroid hypoplasia, therefore, results in an increased M:E ratio with normal appearing hematopoietic precursors. Studies have shown that administration of recombinant erythropoietin will correct the erythroid hypoplasia and may restore the PCV to normal. With prolonged use of human recombinant erythropoietin, veterinary patients may develop antibodies against erythropoietin, resulting in recurrence of red cell hypoplasia and anemia.

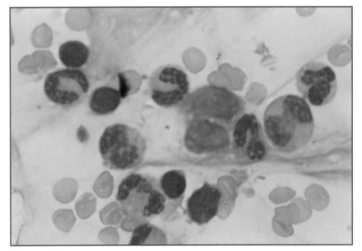

Figure 5. Bone marrow from a cat with renal failure. The sample is of low to normal cellularity and there is a paucity of red cell precursors. The majority of the cells are granulocytic precursors. Several small lymphocytes are present. Note the lack of polychromasia, consistent with a non-regenerative anemia. Wright's stain, 1000X.

CASE 4

SIGNALMENT: Two-year-old castrated male Beagle dog

HISTORY: Fever of unknown origin.

TP	(g/dl)	8.0
PCV	(%)	30
Hb	(g/dl)	10.2
RBC	$(10^{12}/L)$	4.29
MCV	(fl)	70
MCHC	(g/dl)	34
Reticulocytes	$(10^9/L)$	3.5
Platelets	$(10^9/L)$	250.0
WBC	$(10^9/L)$	25.5
Seg. neutrophils	$(10^9/L)$	16.5
Band neutrophils	$(10^9/L)$	2.5
Metamyelocytes	$(10^9/L)$	0.5
Lymphocytes	$(10^9/L)$	2.0
Monocytes	$(10^9/L)$	3.0
Eosinophils	$(10^9/L)$	1.0

HEMOGRAM DESCRIPTION:

Mild normocytic, normochromic anemia in association with a leukocytosis that consists of a neutrophilia with a left shift and a monocytosis.

BONE MARROW EXAMINATION:

The cellularity is high and the M:E ratio is 7.3. Megakaryocytes appear adequate in number and normal in morphology (*Figure 6*). There is a relative increase in myeloid precursors. The erythroid line is decreased in number, but the maturation sequence appears normal. There are approximately 5% lymphocytes and plasma cells seen. Iron stores appear increased (*Figure 7*).

Interpretation

The non-regenerative anemia in conjunction with an inflammatory leukogram is compatible with anemia of chronic disease. This is one of the most common causes of mild to moderate non-regenerative anemia in dogs and cats. In the bone marrow, there is an increase in granulocyte production as part of the inflammatory response. Production of inflammatory mediators results in sequestration of iron, making it less available for red cell production. This sequestration of iron may be appreciated as an increase in hemosiderin or iron stores in a bone marrow sample. Granulocytic hyperplasia together with erythroid hypoplasia results in an increased M:E ratio. The anemia should resolve once the cause of inflammation is eliminated.

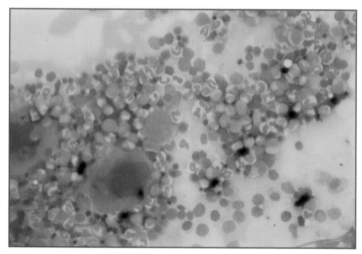

Figure 6. Bone marrow from a dog with anemia of chronic inflammatory disease. Cellularity is very high due to granulocytic hyperplasia. Two normal megakaryocytes are seen. Erythroid precursors are decreased in number and there are increased amounts of hemosiderin. Wright's stain, 200X.

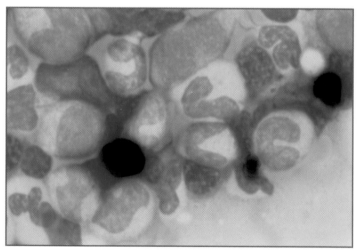

Figure 7. Higher magnification of Figure 6. The maturation of the neutrophilic series is orderly and many bands are seen. The black pigment is hemosiderin. Wright's stain, 1000X.

SIGNALMENT: Eight-year-old castrated male mixed-breed dog

HISTORY: Hyphema and petechiae on mucous membranes.

TP	(g/dl)	8.2
PCV	(%)	14
Hb	(g/dl)	5.1
RBC	(10^{12}/L)	2.04
MCV	(fl)	70
MCHC	(g/dl)	35.5
Reticulocytes	(10^9/L)	8.16
Platelets	(10^9/L)	95.0
WBC	(10^9/L)	16.5
nRBC	(10^9/L)	2.3
Seg. neutrophils	(10^9/L)	11.2
Band neutrophils	(10^9/L)	1.2
Lymphocytes	(10^9/L)	0.3
Monocytes	(10^9/L)	1.2
Eosinophils	(10^9/L)	0.3

HEMOGRAM DESCRIPTION:

Moderate to marked non-regenerative anemia, and a thrombocytopenia. Neutrophils show a left shift, and a lymphopenia is present.

BONE MARROW EXAMINATION:

The M:E ratio is 3.2. There is megakaryocytic and erythroid hypoplasia. The myeloid cell line appears orderly and goes to completion. Dense clusters of well-differentiated plasma cells were seen (*Figure 8*). Hemosiderin is present.

SERUM PROTEIN ELECTROPHORESIS:

There is a hyperproteinemia due to a polyclonal gammopathy and an α-2 spike (*Figure 9*).

Ehrlichia canis titer: 1:10,000

Interpretation

The normocytic, normochromic anemia with lack of reticulocyte response is compatible with a non-regenerative anemia. The presence of bicytopenia (a non-regenerative anemia and thrombocytopenia) warrants examination of the bone marrow. There is hypoplasia of both the megakaryocytic and erythroid cell lines in the bone marrow, suggestive for a primary marrow suppressive disease.

The left shift and lymphopenia suggest possible inflammation with superimposed stress. The mild increase in M:E ratio is likely due to a relative decrease in the erythroid cell line. Although there is a left shift, the neutrophil count is not elevated, making myeloid hyperplasia less likely.

The presence of well-differentiated plasma cells in the bone marrow is also compatible with inflammatory disease and immune stimulation. Multiple myeloma also must be ruled out, as neoplastic plasma cells can appear relatively well differentiated. An inflammatory response is further supported by the serum protein electrophoresis, which demonstrates a polyclonal gammopathy and α-2 spike, compatible with production of antibod-

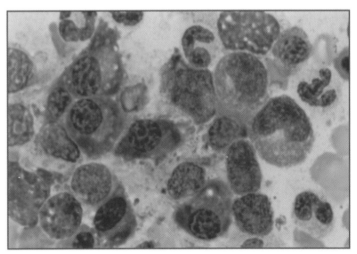

Figure 8. Bone marrow from a dog infected with *E canis* infection. There is a cluster of well-differentiated plasma cells. Maturation of the granulocytic line appears orderly. Several metarubricytes are present, but there is little polychromasia. Wright's stain, 1000X.

ies and acute phase proteins. The very high titer to *E canis* supports a diagnosis of infection with this organism.

Ehrlichia canis is a tick-borne infection that can produce a variety of clinical syndromes. Thrombocytopenia is the most common laboratory change, however, pancytopenia may develop with chronicity. The cytopenias are associated with bone marrow

Continued on next page.

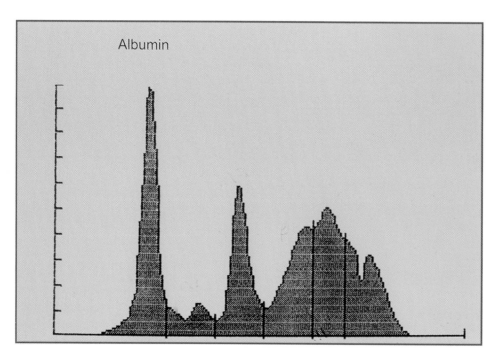

Albumin

Figure 9. Serum protein electrophoresis from a dog infected with *E canis*. The α-2 spike is compatible with inflammation-induced production of acute phase proteins. The wide peak that extends over the beta and gamma region is compatible with polyclonal production of antibodies (polyclonal gammopathy) and also indicates infection.

suppression, as evidenced by marrow hypocellularity. In addition, there is plasma cell hyperplasia in the marrow and hypergammaglobulinemia. The hypergammaglobulinemia is frequently polyclonal, however, monoclonal gammopathies may be observed. Occasionally, *E canis* morula may be seen as inclusions in lymphocytes and mononuclear cells. This is not a reliable means of detecting the organism, and diagnosis usually relies on serology or polymerase chain reaction (PCR) tests.

CASE 6

SIGNALMENT: Three-year-old female mixed-breed dog

HISTORY: Severe rear limb weakness, depression, anorexia, exercise intolerance, and epistaxis within last 10 days.

TP	(g/dl)	8.6
PCV	(%)	34
MCV	(fl)	65
MCHC	(g/dl)	35.5
Reticulocytes	(10^9/L)	none
Platelets	(10^9/L)	180.0
WBC	(10^9/L)	11.2
Seg. neutrophils	(10^9/L)	6.7
Lymphocytes	(10^9/L)	3.2
Monocytes	(10^9/L)	0.5
Eosinophils	(10^9/L)	0.8

HEMOGRAM DESCRIPTION:

Moderate hyperproteinemia and a mild normocytic, normochromic non-regenerative anemia.

SERUM PROTEIN ELECTROPHORESIS:

There is a mild decrease in albumin concentration and a mild increase in the gammaglobulin concentration, which appears to be due to both a polyclonal and a monoclonal gammopathy.

BONE MARROW EXAMINATION:

The cellularity is normal. Megakaryocytes appear adequate. The M:E is 5. Maturation of the myeloid and erythroid series appears orderly and goes to completion. Lymphocytes and plasma cells each are 5% of the nucleated cells. Hemosiderin is present. There are increased numbers of macrophages, some of which contain structures resembling the amastigote stage of *Leishmania infantum* (**Figure 10**).

Interpretation

The mild non-regenerative anemia, mild hypergammaglobulinemia, and mild bone marrow lymphoid and plasma cell hyperplasia are due to chronic inflammation from leishmaniasis. Both polyclonal and monoclonal gammopathies have been reported in dogs with *Leishmania* infections. Leishmaniasis is only rarely reported in dogs in the US and most dogs have traveled to or been imported from endemic areas. This dog had traveled to Greece, which is an endemic area. Leishmaniasis is a multisystemic disease associated with chronic inflammation. The organism is transmitted by sandflies and the incubation period may be months to years.

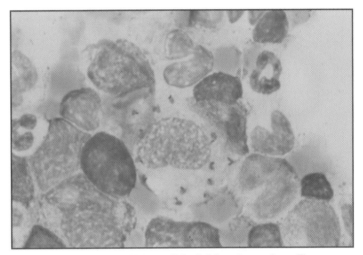

Figure 10. A macrophage with intracellular *Leishmania* organisms. The amastigote forms have a round nucleus and a rod-shaped kinetoplast. Wright's stain, 1000X.

CASE 7

SIGNALMENT: Three-year-old female Domestic Long-haired cat

HISTORY: Anorexia, depression, weight loss, and fever for 3 weeks' duration.

TP	(g/dl)	8.3
PCV	(%)	23
MCV	(fl)	45
MCHC	(g/dl)	34.5
Reticulocytes	(10⁹/L)	none
Platelets	(10⁹/L)	290.0
WBC	(10⁹/L)	24.7
Seg. neutrophils	(10⁹/L)	19.7
Lymphocytes	(10⁹/L)	2.3
Monocytes	(10⁹/L)	2.5
Eosinophils	(10⁹/L)	0.2

HEMOGRAM DESCRIPTION:

Mild hyperproteinemia, mild normocytic, normochromic, non-regenerative anemia, and a mild to moderate leukocytosis due to neutrophilia and monocytosis.

BONE MARROW EXAMINATION:

The cellularity is mildly increased. Megakaryocytes are present in adequate numbers. The M:E is 9.2. Maturation of the myeloid and erythroid series appears orderly and goes to completion. There is mild plasma cell hyperplasia and there are increased numbers of macrophages. Numerous round structures, 2 to 4 microns in diameter are present within the cytoplasm of some macrophages (*Figure 11*). These structures have a basophilic center and a lighter halo around the periphery. The morphology is compatible with the yeast cells of *Histoplasma capsulatum*.

Interpretation

The mild non-regenerative anemia is likely due to anemia of chronic disease. The neutrophilia and monocytosis support a diagnosis of inflammation. The bone marrow aspirate was performed because there was no apparent cause for the fever, anemia, and inflammatory leukogram. The increased M:E likely reflects myeloid hyperplasia and erythroid hypoplasia. The increased numbers of plasma cells and macrophages support a diagnosis of chronic granulomatous inflammation. The etiologic diagnosis is histoplasmosis. Infections occur most commonly in the Ohio, Mississippi, and Missouri river valley region. Clinical findings often are nonspecific or associated with specific organ involvement. For example, cats with histoplasmosis involving the lungs often present for tachypnea and dyspnea.

Cats with histoplasmosis typically have disseminated disease and aspirates from bone marrow, lung, lymph node, or specific sites of inflammation (eg, skin) are recommended for demonstration of the organism. Direct transmission of histoplasmosis from animal to animal or animal to human beings is not reported but concurrent common-source infections have been observed. Fungal cultures that contain the mycelial phase of the organism are highly infectious and should be handled with extreme caution by experienced technologists.

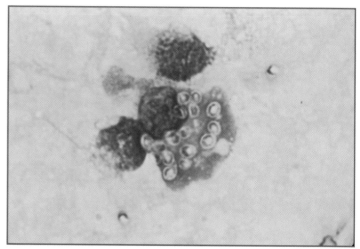

Figure 11. A macrophage with intracellular *Histoplasma* organisms. The yeasts have a round nucleus and a clear halo, which is from shrinkage that occurs during staining. Wright's stain, 1000X.

CASE 8

SIGNALMENT: Seven-year-old intact female Collie dog

HISTORY: Paraparesis, pathologic fractures, and moderately enlarged peripheral lymph nodes.

TP	(g/dl)	7.5
PCV	(%)	47
Hb	(g/dl)	16.5
RBC	(10^{12}/L)	6.7
MCV	(fl)	70
MCHC	(g/dl)	35.0
Platelets	(10^9/L)	352
WBC	(10^9/L)	13.8
Seg. neutrophils	(10^9/L)	10.0
Lymphocytes	(10^9/L)	1.4
Monocytes	(10^9/L)	1.2
Eosinophils	(10^9/L)	1.2

HEMOGRAM DESCRIPTION:

No abnormalities.

PERTINENT BIOCHEMICAL DATA:

There is moderate hypercalcemia (13.9 mg/dl; reference interval = 9.4-12.0 mg/dl).

POPLITEAL LYMPH NODE ASPIRATE:

There is a uniform population of medium to large lymphoid cells with moderately condensed chromatin, an increased amount of moderately basophilic cytoplasm, and inconspicuous nucleoli. Only rare small lymphocytes are present.

BONE MARROW EXAMINATION:

The cellularity appears increased. Only rare megakaryocytes are present. Ninety-one percent of the nucleated cells are immature lymphoid cells with morphologic features similar to those described for the popliteal lymph node aspirate (*Figure 12*). Only rare myeloid and erythroid precursors are present. Maturation of these cells appears orderly and goes to completion. The M:E is 8.0.

Interpretation

Although no abnormalities were detected on the CBC, subsequent review of the blood film by the clinical pathologist revealed rare immature lymphocytes characterized by a medium to large size, moderately condensed chromatin, and an increased amount of moderately basophilic cytoplasm (*Figure 13*). These cells were similar in morphology to those in the lymph node and bone marrow aspirate smears, and were interpreted as neoplastic lymphocytes. About 50% of dogs with lymphoma have circulating neoplastic lymphocytes, based on light microscopic evaluation of blood smears, but the numbers of abnormal cells often is so low that they are not detected in routine evaluation.

Continued on next page.

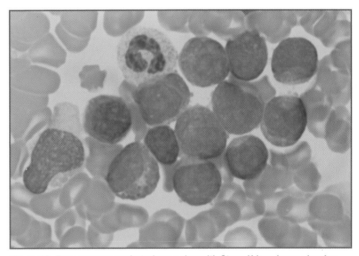

Figure 12. Bone marrow aspirate from a dog with Stage V lymphoma showing marked infiltration with neoplastic lymphocytes. Only rare erythroid and myeloid cells were present. Wright's stain, 1000X.

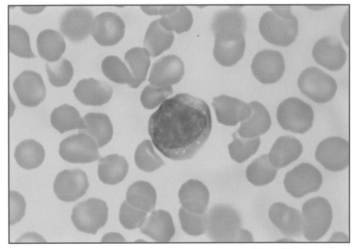

Figure 13. Immature lymphocyte in the peripheral blood. This cell is larger than is typical for normal lymphocytes. The chromatin is finely stippled, a prominent nucleolus is present, and there is abundant basophilic cytoplasm. Wright's stain, 1000X.

The bone marrow aspirate was performed as part of the clinical staging for lymphoma. Bone marrow involvement indicates Stage V lymphoma, which has a worse prognosis than other stages. The morphology of the neoplastic lymphocytes in the lymph node and bone marrow aspirates is typical for lymphoblastic lymphoma. Immunophenotypic analysis has shown that most lymphoblastic lymphomas in dogs are T lymphocytes. Immunophenotyping was not done on this case. Determination of cell lineage may affect prognosis. Dogs with T-cell lymphoma have a worse prognosis than dogs with B-cell lymphoma. Hypercalcemia occurs in some dogs with lymphoma due to increased concentration of parathyroid hormone-related protein (PTH-RP).

CASE 9

SIGNALMENT: Nine-year-old spayed female Golden Retriever dog

HISTORY: Lethargy and anorexia for 2 weeks.

TP	(g/dl)	7.0
PCV	(%)	24
Hb	(g/dl)	8.0
RBC	(10^{12}/L)	3.73
MCV	(fl)	65
MCHC	(g/dl)	33.8
Reticulocytes	(10^9/L)	14.4
Platelets	(10^9/L)	50
WBC	(10^9/L)	99.9
Seg. neutrophils	(10^9/L)	21.0
Lymphocytes	(10^9/L))	65.9
Monocytes	(10^9/L)	13.0

HEMOGRAM DESCRIPTION:

Moderate normocytic, normochromic, non-regenerative anemia; thrombocytopenia; marked leukocytosis due to moderate neutrophilia; moderate monocytosis; and marked lymphocytosis. The majority of the lymphocytes are immature lymphoid cells characterized by a large size; a large, round nucleus; finely stippled nuclear chromatin; 1 to 3 prominent nucleoli; and a moderate amount of basophilic cytoplasm. These cells are interpreted as neoplastic lymphocytes, recognizing that cell lineage frequently cannot be determined by light microscopic evaluation of morphology.

BONE MARROW EXAMINATION:

The cellularity is increased. Rare megakaryocytes and erythroid and myeloid precursors are present. An M:E ratio was not determined due to the presence of too few myeloid and erythroid cells. Ninety percent of the nucleated cells are immature lymphoid cells with a morphologic appearance similar to those seen in the peripheral blood (*Figure 14*).

CYTOCHEMICAL STAINS:

The neoplastic lymphoid cells were negative for CAE, ANBE, and ALP activities.

Interpretation

The non-regenerative anemia, thrombocytopenia, and marked lymphocytosis due the presence of immature lymphoid cells are compatible with hematopoietic neoplasia and the primary differentials would be acute lymphoid leukemia (ALL) and lymphoma. The clinical signs were most compatible with acute lymphoid leukemia. Most dogs with ALL present with vague clinical signs. Most dogs with lymphoma have the multicentric form and present with markedly enlarged peripheral lymph nodes. The hematologic changes also are more compatible with ALL than lymphoma. Dogs with ALL frequently have non-regenerative anemia, neutropenia, thrombocytopenia, or some combination of peripheral cytopenias. Typically, ALL is associated with marked lymphocytosis involving morphologically immature lymphoid cells. This is in contrast to the marked lymphocytosis in dogs with chronic lymphoid leukemia (CLL), in which the cells appear well-differentiated. Dogs with lymphoma may have circulating neoplastic lymphocytes but the numbers of cells are so low that they are often missed in routine evaluation of the blood smear. Cytopenias are not typically present in dogs with lymphoma unless there is marked bone marrow involvement (Stage V lymphoma) or the animal has been given chemotherapy.

Although the clinical signs and hematologic findings were most compatible with a diagnosis of ALL, a bone marrow aspirate was done to confirm the diagnosis. Cytochemical stains were performed to determine cell lineage, since it often is difficult to distinguish myeloblasts from lymphoblasts. The negative staining reaction for CAE, ANBE, and ALP is most compatible with a lymphoid lineage. Presumably very immature myeloblasts could also be negative for these cytochemical stains. More conclusive evidence of lymphoid cell lineage could have been provided by immunophenotyping, but this was not done in this case.

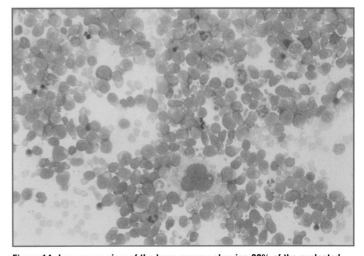

Figure 14. Low power view of the bone marrow showing 90% of the nucleated cells are immature lymphocytes. Rare neutrophils are present for cell size reference. A megakaryocyte is seen in the lower center portion of the figure. Wright's stain, 200X.

SIGNALMENT: Seven-year-old spayed female Golden Retriever dog
HISTORY: Presented for anorexia, lethargy, and icterus.

TP	(g/dl)	8.5
PCV	(%)	47
Hb	(g/dl)	17.7
RBC	(10^{12}/L)	6.86
MCV	(fl)	68
MCHC	(g/dl)	38.0
Platelets	(10^9/L)	244.0
WBC	(10^9/L)	42.3
Seg. neutrophils	(10^9/L)	11.1
Lymphocytes	(10^9/L)	30.0
Monocytes	(10^9/L)	1.2

HEMOGRAM DESCRIPTION:

Moderate hyperproteinemia and marked leukocytosis due to lymphocytosis. The lymphocytes were small and had condensed chromatin.

PERTINENT BIOCHEMICAL DATA:

There was marked hyperbilirubinemia (11.4 mg/dl; reference interval = 0.1-0.5 mg/dl). Liver enzymes were moderately to markedly increased (alanine aminotransferase 204 IU/L; reference interval = 15-110 IU/L; alkaline phosphatase 1200 IU/L; reference interval = 20-130 IU/L).

SERUM PROTEIN ELECTROPHORESIS:

The hyperproteinemia is associated with a monoclonal gammopathy.

BONE MARROW EXAMINATION:

The cellularity appears mildly increased. Megakaryocytes appear adequate. The M:E was 1.0. Maturation of the myeloid and erythroid series appears orderly and goes to completion. Forty percent of the cells are small lymphocytes that resemble those in the peripheral blood (*Figure 15*).

Interpretation

The marked lymphocytosis and relatively mature morphology of the lymphocytes is suggestive of chronic lymphoid leukemia (CLL). Although lymphocytosis may be associated with inflammation, immune mediated disease, or chronic inflammation, non-neoplastic lymphocytoses usually are less than 20,000/µl. Dogs with CLL typically have lymphocyte counts that are greater than 20,000/µl. The bone marrow is infiltrated with neoplastic lymphocytes in dogs with CLL. Spleen and liver also may be involved, as in this dog.

Some dogs with chronic lymphocytic leukemia have subclinical disease. The anorexia, lethargy, icterus, and increased liver enzymes in this dog were due to liver and splenic infiltration with neoplastic lymphocytes. Monoclonal gammopathies occur in about 50% of dogs with CLL. Dogs with subclinical CLL recognized incidentally on routine hemograms often remain stable for months to 1 to 2 years. Dogs with clinical signs and organ infiltration, as were present in this dog, are more likely to have progressive disease, which may terminate in a blast crisis.

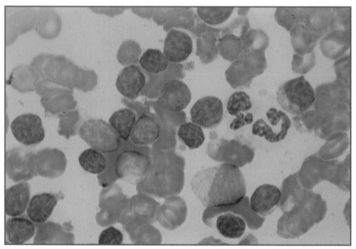

Figure 15. Bone marrow from a dog with chronic lymphoid leukemia. The neoplastic lymphocytes are small and have condensed chromatin, inconspicuous nucleoli, and a scant amount of cytoplasm. Wright's stain, 1000X.

CASE 11

SIGNALMENT: Ten-year-old spayed female mixed-breed dog

HISTORY: Lethargy, pale mucous membranes, and petechiae.

TP	(g/dl)	11.0
PCV	(%)	26
Hb	(g/dl)	8.9
RBC	(10^{12}/L)	3.83
MCV	(fl)	68
MCHC	(g/dl)	34.0
Reticulocytes	(10^9/L)	3.8
Platelets	(10^9/L)	80.0
WBC	(10^9/L)	9.0
Seg. neutrophils	(10^9/L)	7.9
Lymphocytes	(10^9/L)	0.9
Monocytes	(10^9/L)	0.2

HEMOGRAM DESCRIPTION:

Moderate normocytic, normochromic anemia, thrombocytopenia, and lymphopenia.

BONE MARROW EXAMINATION:

The M:E ratio is 3.0. Megakaryocytes are decreased in number. Red cell precursors appear relatively decreased in number, however, the maturation sequence is orderly and goes to completion. The maturation sequence of the myeloid line also is orderly and goes to completion. There are clusters of pleomorphic plasma cells (*Figure 16*). These plasma cells show moderate anisokaryosis and occasional multinucleated cells are seen. Some plasma cells may be classified as Mott cells in that they contain large cytoplasmic inclusions (Russell bodies), compatible with endoplasmic reticulum distended with antibody. Hemosiderin is present.

SERUM PROTEIN ELECTROPHORESIS:

The hyperproteinemia is associated with a monoclonal gammopathy (*Figure 17*).

Interpretation

The normocytic, normochromic anemia without an adequate reticulocyte response is compatible with a non-regenerative anemia. The presence of a bicytopenia warrants examination of the bone marrow. Hypoplasia of the erythroid and megakaryocytic cell lines suggests primary marrow suppression. The mild increase in the M:E ratio is likely due to erythroid hypoplasia, as there is no increase in circulating neutrophils. The presence of abnormal plasma cells, in conjunction with a monoclonal gammopathy, is compatible with multiple myeloma.

Multiple myeloma is often associated with anemia or various cytopenias in conjunction with a monoclonal hypergammaglobu-

Continued on next page.

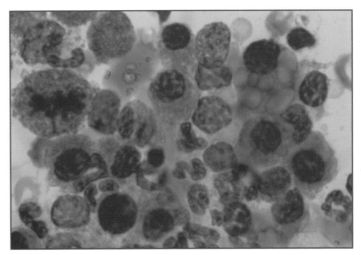

Figure 16. A cluster of neoplastic plasma cells in bone marrow from a dog with multiple myeloma. There is moderate anisocytosis and a mitotic figure is seen. The plasma cell in the upper right corner is a Mott cell that contains multiple Russell bodies (large, pale blue cytoplasmic inclusions). Wright's stain, 1000X.

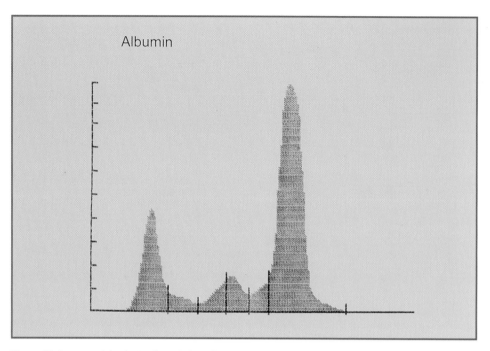

Figure 17. Serum protein electrophoresis from the same dog showing a monoclonal gammopathy.

linemia. The presence of bone lysis may also be associated with a hypercalcemia. Diagnosis of multiple myeloma usually requires the presence of at least 2 of the following: osteolytic lesions, increased plasma cells in the bone marrow (>15%-20% of cells), a monoclonal spike on serum protein electrophoresis, and Bence Jones proteinuria.

CASE 12

SIGNALMENT: Two-year-old female mixed-breed dog

HISTORY: Anorexia and lethargy for 2 weeks.

TP	(g/dl)	6.5
PCV	(%)	30
Hb	(g/dl)	10.6
RBC	(10^{12}/L)	4.38
MCV	(fl)	69
MCHC	(g/dl)	34.5
Platelets	(10^9/L)	180.0
WBC	(10^9/L)	36.0
Seg. neutrophils	(10^9/L)	3.9
Lymphocytes	(10^9/L)	1.8
Monocytes	(10^9/L)	30.3

HEMOGRAM DESCRIPTION:

Mild normocytic, normochromic anemia, and marked leukocytosis due to marked monocytosis. Many of the monocytes appear immature based on finely stippled chromatin, the presence of nucleoli, and increased cytoplasmic basophilia (*Figure 18*).

BONE MARROW EXAMINATION:

Cellularity appears increased. Megakaryocytes appear mildly decreased. The M:E is 2.7. Maturation of the myeloid and erythroid series appears orderly and goes to completion. Lymphocytes and plasma cells are less than 5% of the nucleated cells. Hemosiderin is present. Erythroid cells are less than 50% of the nucleated cells. Sixty percent of all nucleated cells (ANC) are blast cells. The blast cells are characterized by irregularly shaped nuclei, fine chromatin, 1 to 2 nucleoli, and basophilic cytoplasm (*Figure 19*). In some cells, the chromatin appears more reticular, nucleoli are not as prominent, and the cytoplasm appears vacuolated. These cells resemble more mature monocytes. Less than 20% of ANC appear to be granulocytic.

CYTOCHEMICAL STAINING:

The blast cells are negative for CAE activity. Eighty percent of the blast cells are positive for ANBE activity with a diffuse or finely granular pattern (*Figure 20*).

Interpretation

The marked monocytosis is suggestive of monocytic leukemia. Non-neoplastic proliferations of monocytes rarely exceed 10,000/µl. The diagnosis of acute leukemia (AML) was made by first determining that less than 50% of the bone marrow cells were erythroid and then determining that greater than 30% of ANC were blast cells. In this case, the blast cell count includes myeloblasts, monoblasts, and megakaryoblasts and excludes rubriblasts. The diagnosis of acute monocytic leukemia (AML M5) was based on the monocytoid appearance of the more differentiated cells and the diffuse positive staining of the blast cells for ANBE (nonspecific esterase) activity. The AML in this dog most closely resembles M5b because greater than 30%, but less

Continued on next page.

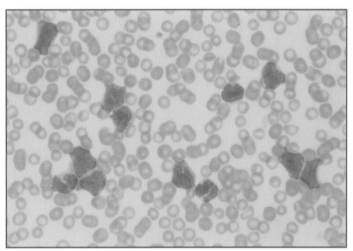

Figure 18. Blood film from a dog with acute monocytic leukemia (AML, M5b) illustrating marked leukocytosis due to the numerous circulating neoplastic monocytes. Wright's stain, 400X.

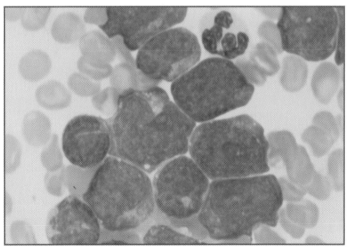

Figure 19. Bone marrow from the same dog. Greater than 30% of ANC were monoblasts. Wright's stain, 1000X.

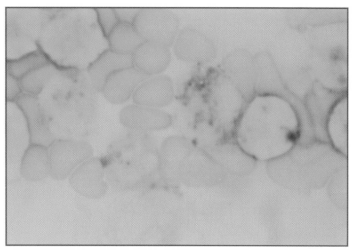

than 80%, of ANC were blasts and there appeared to be differentiation to more mature monocytic cells. AML is rare in dogs. This dog was euthanized due to the poor prognosis of AML.

Figure 20. Bone marrow from the same dog showing the diffuse to finely granular positive staining pattern for ANBE. The monoblast on the right side of the figure has a large positive granule, which is not typical of monocytic cells. ANBE stain, 1000X.

CASE 13

SIGNALMENT: Two-year-old male DSH cat
HISTORY: Lethargy and dyspnea.

TP	(g/dl)	6.7
PCV	(%)	8
Hb	(g/dl)	2.5
RBC	$(10^{12}/L)$	1.14
MCV	(fl)	68
MCHC	(g/dl)	31
Reticulocytes	$(10^9/L)$	6.8
Platelets	$(10^9/L)$	4.0
WBC	$(10^9/L)$	30.3
nRBC	$(10^9/L)$	12.1
Seg. neutrophils	$(10^9/L)$	2.1
Band neutrophils	$(10^9/L)$	1.5
Metamyelocytes	$(10^9/L)$	0.3
Lymphocytes	$(10^9/L)$	3.9
Monocytes	$(10^9/L)$	0.4
Eosinophils	$(10^9/L)$	0.3
Immature cells	$(10^9/L)$	9.7

HEMOGRAM DESCRIPTION:

Multiple cytopenias. A severe macrocytic, normochromic anemia with inadequate reticulocytosis for the severity of the anemia. Also a neutropenia with an orderly left shift and a thrombocytopenia. The majority (40%) of the total nucleated cell count are nucleated red blood cells (nRBC). Many appear to be metarubricytes; however, rubricytes and prorubricytes are also seen. Immature-appearing cells constitute 32% of the nucleated cell count and have characteristics that resemble early erythroid precursors (*Figure 21*). These cells contain a single round nucleus with fine chromatin and occasional nucleoli. Their cytoplasm is deeply basophilic and may contain small vacuoles or fine granules.

BONE MARROW EXAMINATION:

The bone marrow sample is very cellular. Megakaryocytes are absent. The M:E ratio is very low (<0.1) due to a severe hypoplasia of the granulocytic line and a marked increase in erythroid precursors. The maturation sequence of the erythroid line is abnormal with rubriblasts that resemble the immature cells seen on the peripheral blood constituting over 50% of the nucleated cells (*Figure 22*). The erythroid cell line shows some megaloblastic changes as well. Asynchrony of nuclear and cytoplasmic maturation is observed in cells that have immature chromatin patterns in the presence of hemoglobinized cytoplasm. Large metarubricytes are also seen.

Interpretation

This cat has erythroleukemia (M6-Er, formerly erythremic myelosis) secondary to infection with FeLV. The anemia is non-regenerative and there are many circulating nRBCs, but a lack of a reticulocytosis. This may be seen with FeLV infection, in which macrocytosis is not associated with a regenerative response, but rather is due to virus-induced myelodysplasia. The neutropenia and thrombocytopenia may be a consequence of marrow replacement by abnormal red cell precursors as well as direct effects of the virus on these cell lines.

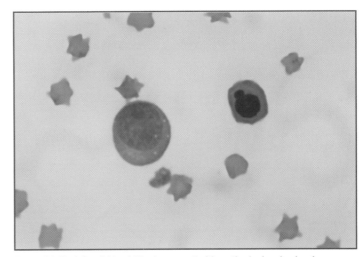

Figure 21. Peripheral blood film from a cat with erythroleukemia showing crenated RBCs, 1 metarubricyte, and 1 immature cell. The metarubricyte has an abnormal nucleus. The immature cell is characterized by a single round nucleus with fine chromatin and deeply basophilic cytoplasm with small vacuoles. Wright's stain, 1000X.

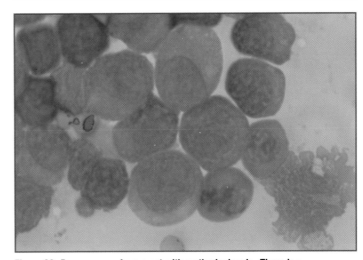

Figure 22. Bone marrow from a cat with erythroleukemia. There is a predominance of immature-appearing erythroblasts. Megaloblastic changes may be seen in the more mature red cell precursors. Wright's stain, 1000X.

CASE 14

SIGNALMENT: Two-year-old male Lhasa Apso dog
HISTORY: Anorexia, weight loss, and intermittent vomiting of several months' duration.

TP	(g/dl)	7.8
PCV	(%)	14
Hb	(g/dl)	4.7
RBC	(10^{12}/L)	1.94
MCV	(fl)	74
MCHC	(g/dl)	33.2
Reticulocytes	(10^9/L)	38.8
Platelets	(10^9/L)	not obtained
WBC	(10^9/L)	38.9
Seg. neutrophils	(10^9/L)	24.1
Band neutrophils	(10^9/L)	3.9
Lymphocytes	(10^9/L)	3.1
Monocytes	(10^9/L)	0.4
Blast cells	(10^9/L)	7.4

HEMOGRAM DESCRIPTION:

Marked normocytic, normochromic non-regenerative anemia, marked leukocytosis due to neutrophilia and a left shift, and circulating blast cells. The blast cells were characterized by conspicuous cytoplasmic blebs, vacuolation, and variable granulation. Macroplatelets had similar cytoplasmic characteristics (*Figure 23*). A platelet count could not be obtained due to many morphologically bizarre macroplatelets.

BONE MARROW EXAMINATION:

The bone marrow was hypercellular. Too few erythroid precursors were present to evaluate maturation; however, myeloid maturation appeared synchronous. No megakaryocytes with normal morphology were observed. Less than 50% of the cells were erythroid. Thirty-three percent of all nucleated cells (ANC) were blast cells. In this case, the blast cell count included myeloblasts, monoblasts, and megakaryoblasts but excluded erythroblasts. The majority of the blast cells were large (20-25 microns in diameter) with round, centrally placed nuclei, finely granular chromatin, and 1 to 3 nucleoli. These cells had a moderate nuclear to cytoplasmic ratio and deeply basophilic cytoplasm that occasionally was granulated and/or vacuolated. Blast cells frequently were binucleate or multinucleate. These multinucleate blast cells varied in size from 30 to 55 microns in diameter and often had abundant, distinctly granular cytoplasm and prominent cytoplasmic blebs (*Figure 24*).

CYTOCHEMICAL STAINING RESULTS:

Blast cells in the bone marrow were negative for SBB and ALP activity. Approximately 33% of the blast cells were weakly positive for ANBE activity. Nearly 100% of the blast cells showed a a coarsely granular pattern when stained for acid phosphatase activity. The acid phosphatase reaction was inhibited with tartrate.

ULTRASTRUCTURAL MORPHOLOGY:

The blast cells had alpha-granules, dense granules, evidence of a developing cytoplasmic demarcation membrane system, and a dilated canalicular system.

FACTOR VIII-RELATED ANTIGEN (von Willebrand's factor):

The blast cells stained intensely positively using indirect immunoperoxidase staining for factor VIII-related antigen.

Interpretation

The presence of primitive-appearing megakaryocytic precursors and megakaryocytic fragments in the circulation, abnormal megakaryocyte morphology, and greater than 30% megakaryoblasts in the bone marrow are most consistent with a diagnosis of acute megakaryoblastic leukemia, which is the M7 classification of acute myeloid leukemia. Dogs with essential thrombocythemia may have morphologically bizarre platelets, but circulating blast cells are absent and blast cells in the bone marrow are less than 30% of ANC. The cytochemical staining pattern and ultrastructural morphology of the blast cells in this dog are consistent with cells of megakaryocytic lineage. The presence of factor VIII-related antigen (von Willebrand's factor) confirms that the blast cells are megakaryoblasts. Megakaryoblastic leukemia is rare in dogs and may occur spontaneously or be associated with radiation exposure. There was no history of radiation exposure in this dog. This dog was euthanized due to a poor prognosis.

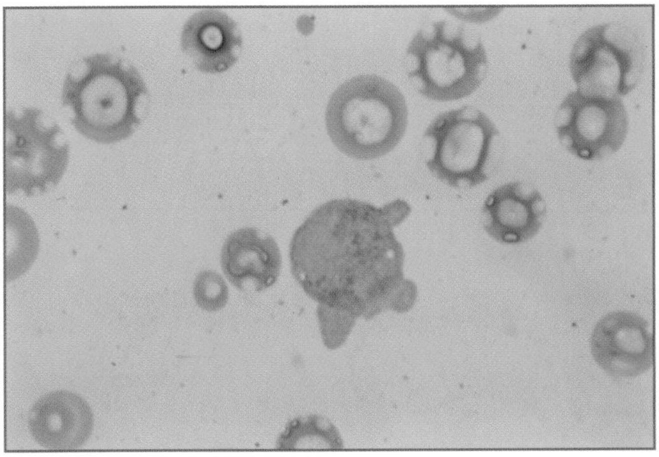

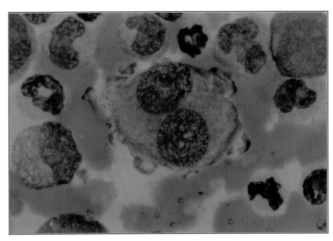

Figure 23. A large platelet with bizarre morphology from a dog with acute megakaryoblastic leukemia (AML, M7). Wright's stain, 1000X. (Blood film courtesy of Dr. Joanne Messick.)

Figure 24. Neoplastic megakaryocyte from the same dog. The binucleate (or multinucleate) morphology is characteristic for neoplastic megakaryocytic cells. Wright's stain, 1000X. (Bone marrow smear courtesy of Dr. Joanne Messick.)

CASE 15

SIGNALMENT: Four-year-old female DSH cat
HISTORY: Anorexia, lethargy, and weakness of 3 days' duration.

TP	(g/dl)	6.4
PCV	(%)	7
Hb	(g/dl)	2.41
RBC	$(10^{12}/L)$	1.26
MCV	(fl)	55.6
MCHC	(g/dl)	34.0
Reticulocytes	$(10^9/L)$	none
Platelets	$(10^9/L)$	not obtained
WBC	$(10^9/L)$	144.2
Seg. neutrophils	$(10^9/L)$	11.5
Lymphocytes	$(10^9/L)$	4.3
Monocytes	$(10^9/L)$	0
Eosinophils (total)	$(10^9/L)$	128.4
Segmented	$(10^9/L)$	50.5
Banded	$(10^9/L)$	5.8
Metamyelocytes	$(10^9/L)$	57.7
Myelocytes	$(10^9/L)$	14.4

HEMOGRAM DESCRIPTION:

Severe macrocytic, normochromic, non-regenerative anemia and marked leukocytosis due to marked eosinophilia. There is a marked left shift in the eosinophils and the eosinophils are poorly granulated (*Figure 25*).

BONE MARROW ASPIRATE:

The cellularity appears mildly increased. Megakaryocytes appear adequate. The M:E is markedly increased because the majority of the cells are immature eosinophils. Eosinophilic precursors include myelocytes, metamyelocytes, and banded forms. Rare cells with bi-lobed or segmented nuclei are present. The immature cells are poorly granulated and difficult to identify as eosinophilic cells. Less than 1% of all nucleated cells (ANC) are blast cells.

CYTOCHEMICAL STAINS:

The eosinophilic cells stained positively for ALP activity, but were negative for SBB, CAE, and ANBE activities.

ULTRASTRUCTURAL MORPHOLOGY:

Electron microscopic examination demonstrated intracytoplasmic crystalline cores typical of feline eosinophil granules.

FELINE LEUKEMIA VIRUS (FeLV) TEST:

Positive.

Interpretation:

The severe macrocytic, non-regenerative anemia could be associated with FeLV infection, the leukemia, or both. The immature cells in the blood and bone marrow were poorly granulated and difficult to recognize as eosinophils; however, the cytochemical staining pattern and ultrastructural morphology are characteristic of eosinophils. Although marked eosinophilia can occur with hypereosinophilic syndrome in cats, the eosinophils are more mature and abnormalities of other blood elements typically are absent. The primary differential diagnosis in this cat was eosinophilic leukemia, based on the marked eosinophilia with a predominance of immature forms. Although less likely, hypereosinophilic syndrome cannot be excluded because less than 30% of ANC were blast cells. This case demonstrates the difficulty in distinguishing between eosinophilic leukemia and hypereosinophilic syndrome. Eosinophilic leukemias in cats are very rare and most cats are FeLV-negative.

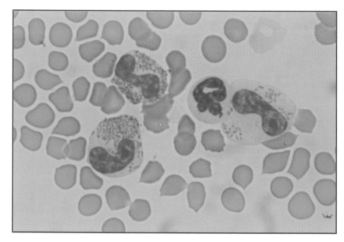

Figure 25. Peripheral blood from a cat with eosinophilic leukemia. There are 3 eosinophils with banded nuclei, 1 of which is poorly granular. Wright's stain, 1000X.

SIGNALMENT: Six-year-old spayed female mixed-breed dog

HISTORY: Presented for lethargy and anorexia with enlarged mesenteric lymph nodes and splenomegaly.

Initial lab results

TP	(g/dl)	6.8
PCV	(%)	31
Hb	(g/dl)	10.4
RBC	(10^{12}/L)	4.69
MCV	(fl)	67
MCHC	(g/dl)	33.3
Reticulocytes	(10^9/L)	not done
Platelets	(10^9/L)	457.0
WBC	(10^9/L)	61.4
nRBC	(10^9/L)	3.1
Seg. neutrophils	(10^9/L)	47.3
Band neutrophils	(10^9/L)	6.1
Lymphocytes	(10^9/L)	1.2
Monocytes	(10^9/L)	2.5
Eosinophils	(10^9/L)	1.2

HEMOGRAM DESCRIPTION:

Mild normocytic, normochromic anemia. There is a marked leukocytosis due to a neutrophilia with a left shift that appears orderly (*Figure 26*).

BONE MARROW EXAMINATION:

The bone marrow is hypercellular and the M:E ratio is 4.0. Megakaryocytes are adequate in number and red cell precursors show orderly maturation. There is an orderly progression in the granulocytic line with 5% promyelocytes, 5% myelocytes, 33% metamyelocytes, 34% bands, and 23% segmented neutrophils (*Figure 27*).

CYTOCHEMICAL STAINS:

Granulocytic precursors stain positive for SBB and CAE. Interestingly, promyelocytes and some myelocytes are positive for ALP, while the metamyelocytes, bands, and segmented neutrophils are negative.

Interpretation

On initial presentation, this hemogram and bone marrow may be interpreted as compatible with inflammatory disease with a mild anemia of chronic disease; however, there was no evidence of inflammatory disease in this dog and she was not febrile at any time. The ALP staining pattern of the granulocyte precursors in the bone marrow was not typical, suggesting a possible myelodysplasia. Normally, granulocytic precursors do not stain with ALP. During subsequent hemograms, the marked leukocytosis persisted. Subsequently, a biopsy of the spleen was taken and the histopathology was compatible with chronic myeloid leukemia (CML). The dog was successfully treated with hydroyurea and remained in remission for 2 years. Variable degrees of leukocytosis were observed when a CBC was periodically repeated.

Two years later, her health progressively declined as she began to have episodes of weakness, anorexia, and lethargy.

Continued on next page.

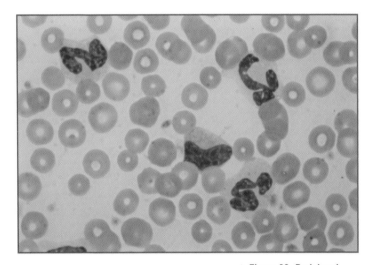

▲ Figure 26. Peripheral blood sample taken from a dog on initial presentation with chronic myeloid leukemia showing an orderly left shift. Wright's stain, 1000X.

Figure 27. Bone marrow ◄ obtained at initial presentation demonstrated an orderly granulocytic hyperplasia. Dysplastic changes were not evident at this time. Wright's stain, 1000X.

Lab results 2 years later:

TP	(g/dl)	6.7
PCV	(%)	10
Hb	(g/dl)	3.4
RBC	(10^{12}/L)	1.27
MCV	(fl)	78
MCHC	(g/dl)	34.7
Reticulocytes	(10^9/L)	15.2
Platelets	(10^9/L)	57.0
WBC	(10^9/L)	42.9
nRBC	(10^9/L)	none
Seg. neutrophils	(10^9/L)	18.1
Band neutrophils	(10^9/L)	9.7
Metamyelocytes	(10^9/L)	5.1
Myelocytes	(10^9/L)	2.5
Blasts	(10^9/L)	4.6
Lymphocytes	(10^9/L)	2.1
Monocytes	(10^9/L)	0.8
Eosinophils	(10^9/L)	none

HEMOGRAM DESCRIPTION:

Marked anemia that is mildly macrocytic, nor-mochromic, and non-regenerative. In addition, there is a thrombocytopenia and macroplatelets were seen. There is a marked leukocytosis with a left shift (*Figure 28*). Circulating blasts are now present and constitute 11% of the cells (*Figure 29*).

CYTOCHEMICAL STAINS:

The mature granulocytes stained positively for SBB and CAE, a normal finding. The blasts were negative for these 2 stains. Occasional blasts were positive for ANBE with a diffuse staining pattern, suggestive for monocytic lineage.

Additional comments:

At the time when the dog came out of remission, her disease had become more aggressive with the appearance of blasts in the circulation. She continued to decline and blasts became more prevalent in subsequent hemograms. She was euthanized after 1 month of unsuccessful therapy.

CML is a rare condition in the dog. The diagnostic dilemma is in distinguishing this condition from a leukemoid reaction or myelodysplastic syndrome. In general, CML is typified by a marked leukocytosis in the absence of inflammation. A disorderly left shift may occur, but there is a lack of overt dysplastic changes in the bone marrow, and toxic changes in the granulocytes are absent.

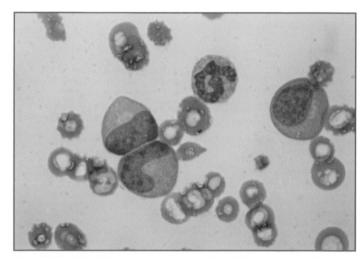

Figure 28. Peripheral blood obtained 2 years after initial presentation. At this time, the disease was no longer in remission and the left shift is less orderly. In addition to the mature segmented neutrophil, there is a band neutrophil, metamyelocyte, and progranulocyte. Note the lack of polychromasia, compatible with a non-regenerative anemia. Wright's stain, 1000X.

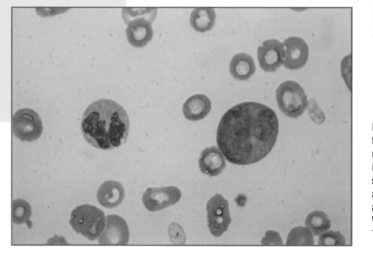

Figure 29. Peripheral blood from the same dog (chronic myeloid leukemia no longer in remission). A mature segmented neutrophil is adjacent to an atypical-appearing monocytoid blast. Wright's stain, 1000X.

CASE 17

Signalment: Six-year-old castrated male cat
History: Gradually progressive exercise intolerance, anorexia, and weight loss.

TP	(g/dl)	6.2
PCV	(%)	6
Hb	(g/dl)	2.0
RBC	$(10^{12}/L)$	1.2
MCV	(fl)	50
MCHC	(g/dl)	33
Reticulocytes	$(10^9/L)$	5.4
Platelets	$(10^9/L)$	4.0
WBC	$(10^9/L)$	3.5
nRBC	$(10^9/L)$	0.2
Seg. neutrophils	$(10^9/L)$	1.3
Lymphocytes	$(10^9/L)$	2.0

HEMOGRAM DESCRIPTION:

Severe normocytic, normochromic, non-regenerative anemia with moderate anisocytosis seen on the slide (*Figure 30*). In addition, there is a marked thrombocytopenia and a leukopenia that consists of a neutropenia and monocytopenia.

BONE MARROW EXAMINATION:

The cellularity of the marrow is low and the M:E ratio is 1.2. Hypoplasia of megakaryocytic, erythroid and myeloid lines is observed. Small lymphocytes constitute 15% of the cells. Histopathologic examination of a core biopsy confirms the cellular hypoplasia and indicates myelofibrosis (*Figure 31*).

FELINE LEUKEMIA VIRUS (FeLV) TEST:

Positive.

Interpretation

The presence of a marked pancytopenia warrants evaluation of a bone marrow. Hypoplasia of both the erythroid and myeloid cell lines results in a normal M:E ratio. Hypoplasia of all cell lines is compatible with primary marrow suppression associated with FeLV infection, which was confirmed by the FeLV test. Myelofibrosis may be one consequence of FeLV infection.

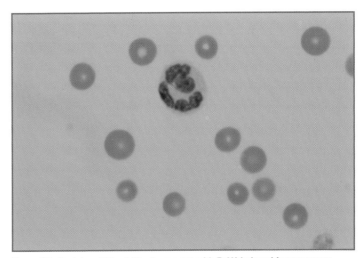

Figure 30. Peripheral blood film from a cat with FeLV-induced bone marrow suppression. There is mild anisocytosis and a lack of polychromasia, compatible with FeLV-associated bone marrow suppression. Wright's stain, 1000X.

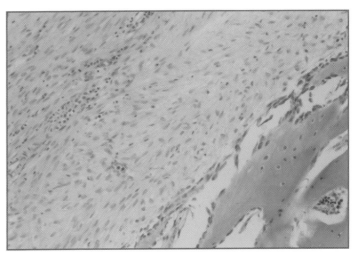

Figure 31. Bone marrow core biopsy from the same cat. There is widespread myelofibrosis and a lack of adequate hematopoietic precursors. H&E stain, 100X.

CASE 18

SIGNALMENT: Nine-year-old male
  Rottweiler dog
HISTORY: Anorexia, lethargy, weight loss,
  pale mucous membranes, and
  splenomegaly.

TP	(g/dl)	5.5
PCV	(%)	18
Hb	(g/dl)	5.9
RBC	$(10^{12}/L)$	2.54
MCV	(fl)	70
MCHC	(g/dl)	33.2
Reticulocytes	$(10^9/L)$	15.2
Platelets	$(10^9/L)$	57.0
WBC	$(10^9/L)$	10.1
nRBC	$(10^9/L)$	0.1
Seg. neutrophils	$(10^9/L)$	7.8
Band neutrophils	$(10^9/L)$	0.2
Lymphocytes	$(10^9/L)$	1.7
Monocytes	$(10^9/L)$	0.2
Eosinophils	$(10^9/L)$	0.1

HEMOGRAM DESCRIPTION:

Marked normocytic, normochromic anemia, and
a thrombocytopenia.

BONE MARROW EXAMINATION:

The bone marrow is hypercellular with an M:E
ratio of 4.3. Maturation sequences of erythroid
and myeloid lines are orderly and go to completion (*Figure 32*). There are moderate numbers of
large, pleomorphic cells with 1 to multiple nuclei
with finely granular chromatin and multiple
nucleoli (*Figure 33*). These cells show marked
anisocytosis and anisokaryosis and multinucleated giant cells were seen. Mitotic figures are common and often bizarre. The cytoplasm of these
cells is abundant, lightly basophilic, and vacuolated. These cells are interpreted as neoplastic
histiocytes. Phagocytosis of erythrocytes by
some of the neoplastic cells is seen.

Interpretation

Malignant histiocytosis is a systemic neoplastic proliferation
of atypical-appearing histiocytes that may occur in dogs and
rarely in cats. In this disease, there are usually one or more
cytopenias observed on the hemogram. In this case, the low TP
in conjunction with an anemia may be due in part to blood loss,
secondary to thrombocytopenia. Liver damage from infiltration
with neoplastic histiocytes may also contribute to low TP.
Phagocytosis of erythrocytes and leukocytes by malignant histiocytes may be marked and is believed to contribute to the peripheral cytopenias. The histiocytic lineage of these cells was confirmed by positive staining with ANBE and lysozyme.

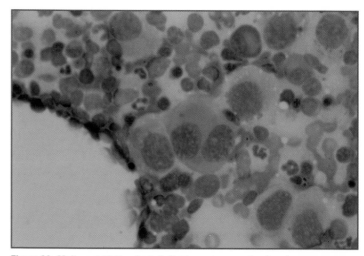

Figure 32. Malignant histiocytosis in the bone marrow of a dog. Large
pleomorphic histiocytes are admixed with granulocytic and erythroid precursors.
Wright's stain, 400X.

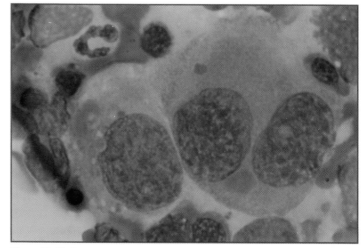

Figure 33. Malignant histiocytes that have phagocytized RBCs. One binucleate
cell is seen. Wright's stain, 1000X.

CASE 19

SIGNALMENT: Ten-year-old spayed female
   Bouvier des Flandres dog
HISTORY: Anorexia, lethargy, and dyspnea
   for 8 days' duration. A mammary mass
   has been present for 4 weeks and recently
   has become inflamed.

TP	(g/dl)	7.3
PCV	(%)	45
Hb	(g/dl)	15.4
RBC	$(10^{12}/L)$	6.9
MCV	(fl)	65
MCHC	(g/dl)	34.6
Platelets	$(10^9/L)$	64.0
WBC	$(10^9/L)$	17.6
Seg. neutrophils	$(10^9/L)$	14.6
Lymphocytes	$(10^9/L)$	1.6
Monocytes	$(10^9/L)$	1.2
Eosinophils	$(10^9/L)$	0.2

HEMOGRAM INTERPRETATION:

Mild leukocytosis due to neutrophilia, and a
moderate thrombocytopenia.

BONE MARROW EXAMINATION:

There are numerous clusters of large, polyhedral
to irregularly shaped cells (*Figure 34*). Features
of anaplasia include large, round to irregularly
shaped nuclei, fine chromatin, and prominent
nucleoli. Numerous mitotic figures are present.
These cells are interpreted as malignant epithelial cells. Only rare megakaryocytes are present
and too few myeloid and erythroid cells are present to determine an M:E ratio or characterize
maturation.

Interpretation

The mild neutrophilia and thrombocytopenia could be due to
the inflamed mammary mass or tumor metastasis to the bone
marrow. The clustering and morphology of the neoplastic cells
suggests an epithelial origin and the anaplastic features are compatible with a malignant neoplasm, which is corroborated by the
metastatic behavior. The mammary mass was an adenocarcinoma
which had metastasized to the lung and bone marrow. Although
the primary neoplasm was evident in this dog, bone marrow aspiration has been shown to be useful in the diagnosis of occult neoplasia in animals with inflammatory leukograms, leukoerythroblastosis, and fever of unknown origin.

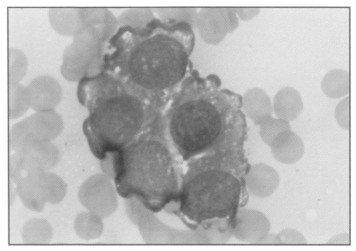

Figure 34. Bone marrow from a dog with metastatic mammary neoplasia. The
cluster of neoplastic cells is typical for malignant glandular epithelial cells.
Wright's stain, 1000X.

	Units	Dog	Cat
Total protein (TP)	g/dl	6.0 - 8.0	6.0 - 8.0
Hematocrit (PCV)	%	37 - 52	25 - 44
Hemoglobin (Hb)	g/dl	12.5 - 19.0	8.5 - 16.0
RBC	$\times 10^{12}$/L	5.5 - 7.5	5.0 - 9.0
MCV	fl	64 - 74	42 - 52
MCHC	g/dL	33.6 - 36.4	31.0 - 35.0
Reticulocytes	$\times 10^9$/L	<60	<60
Platelets	$\times 10^9$/L	150 - 500	150 - 400
Total nucleated cells (WBC)	$\times 10^9$/L	6.5 - 19	4.5 - 16.5
Nucleated RBCs (nRBC)	$\times 10^9$/L	0	0
Segmented neutrophils	$\times 10^9$/L	3.0 - 11.5	3.0 - 13.0
Band neutrophils	$\times 10^9$/L	0 - 0.3	0 - 0.3
Metamyelocytes	$\times 10^9$/L	0	0
Lymphocytes	$\times 10^9$/L	1.2 - 5.2	1.2 - 9.0
Monocytes	$\times 10^9$/L	0.2 - 1.3	0 - 0.7
Eosinophils	$\times 10^9$/L	0 - 1.2	0 - 1.2
Basophils	$\times 10^9$/L	0	0

These reference ranges are from The Ohio State University Clinical Pathology Laboratory. Normal reference ranges vary among other institutions and laboratories.

Index of Figures

Chapter 1

Chapter 3

Chapter 4

Fig. 2.........Bone marrow smear from a dog illustrating numerous blue-staining areas at the base of the smear. These represent spicules or particles of bone and are an indication that an adequate sample was collected. Wright's stain.

Fig. 3.........Hypercellular spicule from a dog with acute myeloid leukemia. Greater than 50% of the spicule is occupied by hematopoietic cells and less than 50% of the spicule is occupied by adipocytes. Wright's stain, 100×.

Fig. 4.........Hypocellular particle from a dog with pancytopenia of undetermined etiology. Less than 30% of the spicule is occupied by hematopoietic cells and more than 70% of the spicule is occupied by adipocytes. Wright's stain, 100×.

Fig. 5.........Megakaryocytes associated with a spicule of bone marrow from a dog with mild megakaryocytic hyperplasia. Typically, 2 to 7 megakaryocytes are present per spicule. There are 9 megakaryocytes associated with this spicule. Megakaryocyte number is easily evaluated with low power magnification because the cells are very large. Wright's stain, 100×.

Fig. 6.........Immature megakaryocyte surrounded by myeloid and erythroid precursors. Notice how much larger the megakaryocytic cell is than the other hematopoietic precursors. The minimal amount of basophilic, agranular cytoplasm is characteristic of immature megakaryocytes. Wright's stain, 400×.

Fig. 7.........Mature megakaryocyte surrounded by myeloid and erythroid precursors. Notice the abundant granular cytoplasm compared to the immature megakaryocyte in the previous figure. Wright's stain, 400×.

Fig. 8.........Myeloid cells from a dog with normal hematopoiesis. Myeloid cells are characterized by round, oval, indented, or segmented nuclei; finely stippled chromatin; and lightly basophilic cytoplasm with primary or secondary granules. Wright's stain, 1000×.

Fig. 9.........Erythroid cells from a dog with normal hematopoiesis. Erythroid cells are characterized by round nuclei, condensed chromatin, and basophilic, agranular cytoplasm. Wright's stain, 1000×.

Fig. 10.......Schematic of myeloid to erythroid (M:E) ratios. Myeloid cells are indicated by the white circles and erythroid cells are indicated by the red circles. The normal M:E ratio is 0.75 to 2.5 in dogs and 1.0 to 3.0 in cats. The illustration depicts normal, decreased, and increased M:E ratios, and mechanisms associated with each kind of change. Examples of diseases that might be associated with each type of mechanism are indicated in red. (Illustration by Tim Vojt.)

Fig. 11.......Schematic representation of maturation of myeloid and erythroid precursors showing the "pyramid" effect of very few immature precursors forming the apex of the pyramid and numerous differentiated cells forming the base of the pyramid. This is an indication of orderly maturation that progresses to completion. (Illustration by Tim Vojt.)

Fig. 12.......Bone marrow from a dog with normal hematopoiesis showing two segmented neutrophils, 1 metarubricyte, 1 rubricyte, and 2 small lymphocytes. Lymphocytes have a higher nuclear to cytoplasmic ratio, less condensed chromatin, and lighter staining cytoplasm than metarubricytes. The lymphocyte in the upper left is broken but a narrow rim of cytoplasm can be seen on the left side of the lymphocyte on the lower left. A metarubricyte is located between these 2 lymphocytes. Wright's stain, 1000×.

Fig. 13.......Plasma cells from the bone marrow of a dog with plasma cell hyperplasia. Plasma cells are large, round to oval cells with abundant basophilic cytoplasm and an eccentrically placed nucleus. There often is a perinuclear clear zone, which is very prominent in the plasma cells shown here. This likely represents the Golgi area. Wright's stain, 1000×.

Fig. 14.......A Mott cell from the bone marrow of a dog with plasma cell hyperplasia. The round, pale structures are called Russell bodies, and likely represent rough endoplasmic reticulum distended with antibody. Wright's stain, 1000×.

Fig. 15.......Two macrophages distended with hemosiderin are shown in this figure. Occasional macrophages are present in bone marrow smears from healthy animals but they may be difficult to recognize unless they have phagocytized cells or etiologic agents or contain pigment granules, as shown here. Wright's stain, 1000×.

Fig. 16.......A spicule of bone marrow from a dog with myeloid and erythroid hyperplasia. The clear spaces associated with the spicule represent the cytoplasm of adipocytes. The nucleus often is difficult to visualize. Wright's stain, 100×.

Fig. 17.......An osteoclast from a dog with normal hematopoiesis. Osteoclasts are recognized infrequently. Like megakaryocytes, they are very large cells with abundant cytoplasm, but osteoclasts have multiple nuclei that appear separated from each other, in contrast to the multilobed nuclei in megakaryocytes. The cytoplasmic granules present in this cell sometimes are seen in osteoclasts and these are much larger than the granules in megakaryocytes. Wright's stain, 1000×.

Fig. 18.......An aggregate of endothelial cells from part of a small blood vessel. Endothelial cells are characterized by their elongated shape and narrow nucleus. Wright's stain, 400×.

Fig. 19.......Two mast cells and 2 neutrophils from a cat with mast cell leukemia. Mast cells are recognized by their prominent cytoplasmic granules, which stain purple with Wright's stain. The round nucleus may be obscured if the granules are numerous. 1000×.

Fig. 20.......A spicule of bone marrow with abundant hemosiderin, which appears as dark greenish black granules. Hemosiderin is an iron-protein complex that is stored in macrophages as a source of iron for erythropoiesis. Wright's stain, 1000×.

Fig. 21.......A core biopsy from a normal dog illustrating approximately 50% cellularity. H&E stain, 100×.

Fig. 22.......A core biopsy from a normal dog showing hematopoietic elements interspersed with fat. Two mature megakaryocytes are seen and are the largest of the blood forming elements. Iron stores may be seen as brown pigment. H&E stain, 400×.

Chapter 5

Fig. 1.........Erythroid hyperplasia in a dog with immune-mediated hemolytic anemia. There is a relative increase in prorubricytes and rubricytes. One mitotic figure (upper left) and marked polychromasia is seen. Wright's stain, 1000×.

Fig. 2.........Granulocytic hyperplasia in a dog. There is a relative increase in progranulocytes and myelocytes, and a decrease in band and mature segmented neutrophils (left shift). Wright's stain, 1000×.

Fig. 3.........Bone marrow from a dog with granulocytic hyperplasia with a left shift due to inflammation. Anemia of chronic inflammatory disease has developed and is characterized by erythroid hypoplasia and an increase in iron stores, seen as an increase in hemosiderin. Wright's stain, 400×.

Fig. 4.........A cluster of monocytic precursors in the bone marrow of a dog. Wright's stain, 1000×.

Fig. 5.........Megakaryocytic hyperplasia in a dog with immune-mediated thrombocytopenia. Particles contain increased numbers of megakaryocytes at various developmental stages. Wright's stain, 200×.

Fig. 6. ......A cluster of well-differentiated plasma cells in the bone marrow of a dog with chronic inflammatory disease. Granulocytic hyperplasia is also evident. Wright's stain, 400×.

Fig. 7.........A core biopsy of bone marrow from a dog with aplastic anemia. The bone marrow contains fat and small blood vessels, but no hematopoietic precursors are evident. H&E, 200×.

Fig. 8.........Bone marrow from a dog with immune-mediated hemolytic anemia. There is generalized hyperplasia of the marrow with increases in both erythroid and granulocytic precursors (consequently a normal M:E). The maturation sequences of the hematopoietic precursors are orderly, with many metarubricytes as well as band and segmented neutrophils seen. Wright's stain, 400×.

Fig. 9.........Bone marrow from a dog with IHA illustrating phagocytosis of early red cell precursors by macrophages. Wright's stain, 400×.

Fig. 10.......Bone marrow from a dog with inflammatory disease. Cytoplasmic vacuolation is seen as part of toxic changes in the granulocytic precursors. Wright's stain, 1000×.

Fig. 11.......Histiocytic hyperplasia with marked erythrophagocytosis present in a dog with hemophagocytic syndrome. Two morphologically normal macrophages are seen, one of which contains phagocytized RBCs and hemosiderin. In addition, there is granulocytic hyperplasia, compatible with inflammatory disease. Wright's stain, 1000×.

Fig. 12.......*Mycobacteria* organisms from a dog with systemic infection. The organisms appear as unstained rods, 0.2 to 0.5 microns wide and 1.0 to 3.0 microns long and most often are located within macrophages. Acid-fast staining is recommended for presumptive diagnosis. Wright's stain, 1000×.

Fig. 13.......Two macrophages with intracellular *Leishmania* organisms from a dog with systemic Leishmaniasis. This dog had traveled to Greece, which is an endemic area. The amastigote stage of the organism is oval to round, 2.5 to 5 microns long and 1.5 to 2.0 microns wide. A roundish nucleus and a characteristic rod-shaped kinetoplast typically are present. Wright's stain, 1000×.

Fig. 14.......Macrophage containing a schizont of *Cytauxzoon felis*. Infected macrophages can be found in aspirates from bone marrow, spleen, or lymph nodes. The piroplast stage may be seen in RBCs in peripheral blood. Wright's stain, 1000×.

Fig. 15.......A RBC with 2 piriform shaped *Babesia canis* organisms. Parasitized erythrocytes may be seen in peripheral blood and in tissue aspirates from the bone marrow or spleen. Wright's stain, 1000×.

Fig. 16.......A RBC with a chain of *Haemobartonella* organisms is shown in the center left. *H canis* more often forms chains of organisms than does *H felis*. Wright's stain, 1000×.

Fig. 17.......A macrophage with numerous intracellular *Histoplasma* organisms from a cat with systemic infection. The organisms are 2.0 to 4.0 microns in diameter and have a basophilic center with a light halo. Wright's stain, 1000×.

Fig. 18.......Blood film from a dog with iron deficiency is characterized by anisocytosis and marked hypochromasia. Wright's stain, 1000×.

Fig. 19.......Bone marrow from the same dog with iron deficiency. There are decreased numbers of metarubricytes and a relative increase in rubricytes. Some asynchrony in nuclear and cytoplasmic maturation is evident with clumping of chromatin out pacing hemoglobinization of the cells. Wright's stain, 1000×.

Fig. 20.......Megaloblastic changes observed in the bone marrow from a cat with myelodysplastic disease secondary to FeLV infection. There is asynchrony of nuclear and cytoplasmic maturation evident within the red cell precursors, which contain large, immature nuclei with fine chromatin and nucleoli, but hemoglobinized and granular cytoplasm. Wright's stain, 1000×.

Chapter 6

Fig. 21.......Neoplastic mast cells from a cat with mast cell leukemia. Mast cells are characterized by the presence of numerous purple cytoplasmic granules. Wright's stain, 1000×.

Fig. 22.......Neoplastic mast cells from a dog with systemic mastocytosis. These mast cells are very anaplastic based on marked variation in cell size, nuclear size, and nuclear to cytoplasmic ratio, and minimal granularity. Wright's stain, 1000×.

Fig. 23.......Malignant histiocytes from a dog with malignant histiocytosis. These cells are characterized by their large size and abundant cytoplasm. There is moderate to marked variation in cell size and nuclear size. Wright's stain, 1000×.

Fig. 24.......Malignant histiocytes from a dog with malignant histiocytosis. These cells have phagocytized erythroid precursors. Wright's stain, 1000×.

Fig. 25.......A cluster of metastatic epithelial cells from a dog with a mammary adenocarcinoma. The acinar formation shown by the cells in the upper left is typical of neoplastic glandular epithelial cells. Wright's stain, 1000×.

Chapter 7

Fig. 1.........Peripheral blood from a dog with IHA and ITP. There is marked anisocytosis and polychromasia. Spherocytes are present. In the center is a macroplatelet. Wright's stain, 1000×.

Fig. 2.........A particle of bone marrow from the same dog with IHA and ITP. The particle is very cellular and there is generalized hyperplasia of the marrow. Megakaryocytic hyperplasia is prominent. Hemosiderin may be seen as black staining material within the cluster of cells. Wright's stain, 1000×.

Fig. 3.........Bone marrow from a dog with hemophagocytic syndrome. There are increased numbers of well-differentiated histiocytes. These macrophages appear actively phagocytic. Wright's stain, 400×.

Fig. 4.........Higher power view of Figure 3. Granulocytic myelocytes and a mitotic figure are seen. The histiocyte in the center of the field has phagocytized several RBCs and platelets. Wright's stain, 1000×.

Fig. 5.........Bone marrow from a cat with renal failure. The sample is of low to normal cellularity and there is a paucity of red cell precursors. The majority of the cells are granulocytic precursors. Several small lymphocytes are present. Note the lack of polychromasia, consistent with a non-regenerative anemia. Wright's stain, 1000×.

Fig. 6.........Bone marrow from a dog with anemia of chronic inflammatory disease. Cellularity is very high due to granulocytic hyperplasia. Two normal megakaryocytes are seen. Erythroid precursors are decreased in number and there are increased amounts of hemosiderin. Wright's stain, 200×.

Fig. 7.........Higher magnification of Figure 6. The maturation of the neutrophilic series is orderly and many bands are seen. The black pigment is hemosiderin. Wright's stain, 1000×.

Fig. 8.........Bone marrow from a dog infected with *E canis* infection. There is a cluster of well-differentiated plasma cells. Maturation of the granulocytic line appears orderly. Several metarubricytes are present, but there is little polychromasia. Wright's stain, 1000×.

Fig. 9.........Serum protein electrophoresis from a dog infected with E canis. The α-2 spike is compatible with inflammation-induced production of acute phase proteins. The wide peak that extends over the beta and gamma region is compatible with polyclonal production of antibodies (polyclonal gammopathy) and also indicates infection.

Fig. 10.......A macrophage with intracellular *Leishmania* organisms. The amastigote forms have a round nucleus and a rod-shaped kinetoplast. Wright's stain, 1000×.

Fig. 11.......A macrophage with intracellular *Histoplasma* organisms. The yeasts have a round nucleus and a clear halo, which is from shrinkage that occurs during staining. Wright's stain, 1000×.

Fig. 12.......Bone marrow aspirate from a dog with Stage V lymphoma showing marked infiltration with neoplastic lymphocytes. Only rare erythroid and myeloid cells were present. Wright's stain, 1000×.

Fig. 13.......Immature lymphocyte in the peripheral blood. This cell is larger than is typical for normal lymphocytes. The chromatin is finely stippled, a prominent nucleolus is present, and there is abundant basophilic cytoplasm. Wright's stain, 1000×.

Fig. 14.......Low power view of the bone marrow showing 90% of the nucleated cells are immature lymphocytes. Rare neutrophils are present for cell size reference. A megakaryocyte is seen in the lower center portion of the figure. Wright's stain, 200×.

Fig. 15.......Bone marrow from a dog with chronic lymphoid leukemia. The neoplastic lymphocytes are small and have condensed chromatin, inconspicuous nucleoli, and a scant amount of cytoplasm. Wright's stain, 1000×.

Fig. 16.......A cluster of neoplastic plasma cells in bone marrow from a dog with multiple myeloma. There is moderate anisocytosis and a mitotic figure is seen. The plasma cell in the upper right corner is a Mott cell that contains multiple Russell bodies (large, pale blue cytoplasmic inclusions). Wright's stain, 1000×.

Fig. 17.......Serum protein electrophoresis from the same dog showing a monoclonal gammopathy.

Fig. 18.......Blood film from a dog with acute monocytic leukemia (AML, M5b) illustrating marked leukocytosis due to the numerous circulating neoplastic monocytes. Wright's stain, 400×.

Fig. 19.......Bone marrow from the same dog. Greater than 30% of ANC were monoblasts. Wright's stain, 1000×.

Fig. 20.......Bone marrow from the same dog showing the diffuse to finely granular positive staining pattern for ANBE. The monoblast on the right side of the figure has a large, positive granule, which is not typical of monocytic cells. ANBE stain, 1000×.

Fig. 21.......Peripheral blood film from a cat with erythroleukemia showing crenated RBCs, 1 metarubricyte and 1 immature cell. The metarubricyte has an abnormal nucleus. The immature cell is characterized by a single round nucleus with fine chromatin and deeply basophilic cytoplasm with small vacuoles. Wright's stain, 1000×.

Fig. 22.......Bone marrow from a cat with erythroleukemia. There is a predominance of immature-appearing erythroblasts. Megaloblastic changes may be seen in the more mature red cell precursors. Wright's stain, 1000×.

Fig. 23.......A large platelet with bizarre morphology from a dog with acute megakaryoblastic leukemia (AML, M7). Wright's stain, 1000×. (Blood film courtesy of Dr. Joanne Messick.)

Fig. 24.......Neoplastic megakaryocyte from the same dog. The binucleate (or multinucleate) morphology is characteristic for neoplastic megakaryocytic cells. Wright's stain, 1000×. (Bone marrow smear courtesy of Dr. Joanne Messick.)

Fig. 25.......Peripheral blood from a cat with eosinophilic leukemia. There are 3 eosinophils with banded nuclei, 1 of which is poorly granular. Wright's stain, 1000×.

Fig. 26.......Peripheral blood sample taken from a dog on initial presentation with chronic myeloid leukemia showing an orderly left shift. Wright's stain, 1000×.

Fig. 27.......Bone marrow obtained at initial presentation demonstrated an orderly granulocytic hyperplasia. Dysplastic changes were not evident at this time. Wright's stain, 1000×.

Fig. 28.......Peripheral blood obtained 2 years after initial presentation. At this time, the disease was no longer in remission and the left shift is less orderly. In addition to the mature segmented neutrophil, there is a band neutrophil, metamyelocyte, and progranulocyte. Note the lack of polychromasia, compatible with a non-regenerative anemia. Wright's stain, 1000×.

Fig. 29.......Peripheral blood from the same dog (chronic myeloid leukemia no longer in remission). A mature segmented neutrophil is adjacent to an atypical-appearing monocytoid blast. Wright's stain, 1000×.

Fig. 30.......Peripheral blood film from a cat with FeLV-induced bone marrow suppression. There is mild anisocytosis and a lack of polychromasia, compatible with FeLV-associated bone marrow suppression. Wright's stain, 1000×.

Fig. 31.......Bone marrow core biopsy from the same cat. There is widespread myelofibrosis and a lack of adequate hematopoietic precursors. H&E stain, 100×.

Fig. 32.......Malignant histiocytosis in the bone marrow of a dog. Large pleomorphic histiocytes are admixed with granulocytic and erythroid precursors. Wright's stain, 400×.

Fig. 33.......Malignant histiocytes that have phagocytized RBCs. One binucleate cell is seen. Wright's stain, 1000×.

Fig. 34.......Bone marrow from a dog with metastatic mammary neoplasia. The cluster of neoplastic cells is typical for malignant glandular epithelial cells. Wright's stain, 1000×.

Glossary of Terms

-A-

Acute myeloid leukemia (AML): Neoplastic transformation of myeloid precursors. In this case, the term myeloid refers to progeny of the multipotential myeloid stem cell, which include granulocytic, monocytic, megakaryocytic, and erythroid precursors.

Acute lymphoid leukemia (ALL): Neoplastic transformation of lymphoid precursors, which could involve B lymphocytes, T lymphocytes, or natural killer (NK) cells.

Acute lymphoid leukemia (ALL): A neoplastic proliferation of lymphoid cells which usually involves a morphologically immature lymphocyte. ALL is characterized by an acute clinical course.

All nucleated cells (ANC): A term used in the classification scheme for acute myeloid leukemia and includes all nucleated cells in the bone marrow except lymphocytes, macrophages, plasma cells, or mast cells.

-B-

Band(ed) neutrophil (or eosinophil): A granulocyte with a nucleus that has parallel sides all around or has a nuclear indentation that is less than a third of the width of the nucleus.

Bicytopenia: A decrease in 2 cell types in the peripheral blood.

Burst-forming unit erythroid (BFU-E): The earlier stage *in vitro* counterpart of erythroid precursors.

Burst-forming unit megakaryocyte (BFU-Meg): The earlier stage *in vitro* counterpart of megakaryocyte precursors.

-C-

Cellularity: The relative ratio of hematopoietic cells to adipocytes in the bone marrow. Normally, 30% to 50% of a bone marrow spicule is occupied by hematopoietic cells and 50% to 70% is occupied by adipocytes.

Chronic lymphoid leukemia (CLL): A neoplastic proliferation of lymphoid cells that usually involves a morphologically mature lymphocyte. CLL is characterized by a chronic clinical course, and initially most animals are not clinically ill.

Chronic myeloid leukemia (CML): A very rarely recognized type of leukemia in dogs and cats. There is a neoplastic proliferation of granulocytic cells that usually maintain the ability to differentiate to mature neutrophils. CML often is a diagnosis of exclusion when other more common causes of marked neutrophilia have been ruled out and the neutrophilia persists for months or years.

Colony-forming unit erythroid (CFU-E): The later stage *in vitro* counterpart of erythroid precursors.

Colony-forming unit blast (CFU-Blast): The *in vitro* counterpart of the pluripotential hematopoietic stem cell.

Colony-forming unit granulocyte-erythrocyte-monocyte-megakaryocyte (CFU-GEMM): The *in vitro* counterpart of the committed myeloid progenitor cell.

Colony-forming unit granulocyte macrophage (CFU-GM): The *in vitro* counterpart of progenitors that develop into granulocytic and monocytic precursors.

Colony-forming unit granulocyte (CFU-G): The *in vitro* counterpart of neutrophil precursors.

Colony-forming unit macrophage (CFU-M): The *in vitro* counterpart of monocyte/macrophage precursors.

Colony-forming unit eosinophil (CFU-Eos): The *in vitro* counterpart of eosinophil precursors.

Colony-forming unit basophil/mast cell (CFU-Baso/Mast): The *in vitro* counterpart of basophil and mast cell precursors. There is some controversy about whether basophils and mast cells share a common progenitor.

Colony-forming unit megakaryocyte (CFU-Meg): The later stage *in vitro* counterpart of megakaryocyte precursors.

Cyclic hematopoiesis: A syndrome of cyclic fluctuations in blood cell counts that has been described in Gray Collie dogs and in cats infected with feline leukemia virus (FeLV).

-D-

Dysplasia: Abnormal hematopoiesis recognized as morphologic abnormalities in the precursors of the affected cell line.

-E-

Erythropoiesis: The production of erythrocytes from erythroid progenitor cells.

Erythropoietin: A hormone secreted by renal peritubular interstitial cells that stimulates erythropoiesis.

Essential thrombocythemia (ET): A type of chronic myeloproliferative disorder that is characterized by persistent, marked thrombocytosis in the absence of physiologic or reactive causes of thrombocytosis. Platelet counts often are in excess of $1,000,000/\mu l$.

-H-

Hemophagocytic syndrome: A non-neoplastic proliferation of macrophages associated with infectious, metabolic, or neoplastic diseases. The macrophages appear normal morphologically.

Hematopoiesis: The process by which undifferentiated stem cells develop into terminally differentiated cells.

Hemosiderin: The storage form of iron in bone marrow macrophages, which appears as dark brownish-green granules with Wright's stain.

-L-

Leukemia: A neoplastic proliferation of hematopoietic cells that originates in the bone marrow. Leukemias often are classified by cell lineage, as myeloid or lymphoid, or by clinical course, as chronic or acute.

Leukemoid reaction: A marked increase in neutrophil counts, which often is associated with a left shift. Neutrophil counts usually are greater than $75,000/\mu l$ in dogs or $50,000/\mu l$ in cats. These counts represent non-neoplastic proliferation of neutrophils.

Leukoerythroblastic reaction: An inappropriate increase in nucleated red blood cells (nRBCs) and immature neutrophils that often indicates primary bone marrow disease. A leukoerythroblastic reaction is an indication for a bone marrow aspirate.

Lymphoma: The malignant transformation of lymphoid cells that originates in tissues other than the bone marrow. The bone marrow may become infiltrated in Stage V lymphoma.

Lymphopoiesis: The development of B lymphocytes, T lymphocytes, and natural killer (NK) cells from lymphoid progenitor cells. Lymphopoiesis occurs in the bone marrow, but maturation of many lymphoid cells occurs in the peripheral lymphoid tissues.

-M-

Malignant histiocytosis: A neoplastic proliferation of histiocytic cells that often involves the bone marrow.

Maturation arrest: A disruption of differentiation at the most terminal stages for a particular cell type. An apparent maturation arrest can occur when there is depletion of the storage pool of granulocytes from rapid peripheral destruction.

Mean corpuscular volume (MCV): The mean volume of RBCs measured in femtoliters (fl). This value is used to determine if RBCs are microcytic, normocytic, or macrocytic, which is part of the classification scheme for anemia.

Mean corpuscular hemoglobin concentration (MCHC): The mean hemoglobin concentration (grams) in a specific volume of RBCs (deciliter). This value (expressed in g/dl) is used to determine if RBCs are normochromic or hypochromic, which is part of the classification scheme for anemia.

Megakaryoblasts: The earliest morphologically recognizable cell for megakaryocyte production. These cells are large and have 1, 2, or 4 nuclei and a minimal amount of intensely basophilic, agranular cytoplasm.

Megakaryocytes: The most mature megakaryocytic cell. Megakaryocytes are very large cells with multilobed nuclei and abundant, granular cytoplasm. Platelets are produced from megakaryocyte.

Megakaryocytopoiesis: The production of megakaryocytes from megakaryocytic progenitor cells.

Megaloblastic cells: Asynchronous maturation of the nucleus and cytoplasm. Megaloblastic changes in erythroid cells are characterized by large, immature nuclei in erythroid cells with fully hemoglobinated cytoplasm and have been observed in vitamin B_{12} deficiency in Giant Schnauzer dogs and in some cats infected with feline leukemia virus (FeLV).

Metamyelocyte: A granulocyte precursor with an indented nucleus and secondary granules.

Metarubricyte: The most mature nucleated erythroid cell. It has a small nucleus with very condensed chromatin. The tinctorial quality of the cytoplasm depends on the concentration of hemoglobin.

Mott cell: A plasma cell with abundant Russell body inclusions.

Multiple myeloma: A neoplastic proliferation of plasma cells that originates in the bone marrow and involves multiple bones.

Myeloblast: The most immature granulocyte precursor that is morphologically recognizable in the bone marrow. It is a large cell with fine chromatin, a prominent nucleolus, and a moderate amount of moderately basophilic cytoplasm.

Myelocyte: A granulocyte precursor characterized by a round nucleus and the initiation of secondary granule formation.

Myelodysplasia (MDS): Abnormal hematopoiesis characterized by peripheral cytopenia and hypercellular bone marrow. Blast cells are increased but less than 30% of ANC or non-erythroid cells. Morphologic abnormalities in multiple cell lines frequently are present.

Myelofibrosis: A histologic term to indicate increased collagen in the bone marrow.

Myeloid: A term sometimes used to refer to the bone marrow (eg, multiple myeloma involves multiple bone marrow sites). It also is used to refer to non-lymphoid cells, in which case it includes granulocytes, monocytes, megakaryocytes, and erythroid cells (eg, myeloid leukemia). The term "myeloid" as the numerator in the M:E ratio refers to only granulocytes and monocytes.

Myeloid to erythroid (M:E) ratio: A numerical estimate of the relative numbers of myeloid (granulocyte and monocyte) precursors and erythroid (RBC) precursors. Certain diseases may be associated with specific changes in the M:E ratio.

Myelophthisis: Marked infiltration of the bone marrow by neoplastic or inflammatory cells, to the exclusion of normal hematopoietic cells. Myelophthisis can occur with hematopoietic neoplasia, metastatic neoplasia, or granulomatous inflammation.

Myelopoiesis: The production of granulocytes and monocytes from myeloid progenitor cells.

-N-

Natural killer (NK) cells: Non-T, non-B lymphoid cells that can lyse tumor cells, virally-infected cells, and some normal cells, without prior sensitzation.

Non-erythroid cells (NEC): A term used in the classification scheme for acute myeloid leukemia and is calculated from all nucleated cells (ANC) minus all erythroid cells.

-P-

Packed cell volume (PCV): The volume of blood that is due to red blood cells, measured as a percentage. Usually, PCV can be used interchangeably with hematocrit. PCV is the most commonly used parameter in veterinary medicine to determine if an animal is anemic.

Pancytopenia: A decrease in RBCs, leukocytes, and platelets in the peripheral blood.

Polycythemia vera (PV): Primary polycythemia; a form of chronic myelogenous leukemia in which there is a persistently increased RBC mass in the presence of normal oxygen saturation and normal or low serum erythropoietin.

Precursor cells: Morphologically recognizable hematopoietic cells that develop from lineage specific progenitors and mature into lineage restricted terminally differentiated cells. For example, myeloblasts, progranulocytes, myelocytes, and metamyelocytes are neutrophil precursors.

Primary granules: The azurophilic granules that form at the progranulocyte stage of development of myeloid cells.

Primary polycythemia: *See Polycythemia vera (PV).*

Progenitor cells: Cells that have little if any capacity for self-renewal and are committed to cell production along a limited number of lineages. Lymphoid progenitor cells differentiate into B lymphocytes, T lymphocytes, and natural killer (NK) cells. Myeloid progenitor cells differentiate into granulocytes, monocytes, megakaryocytes, and erythrocytes.

Progranulocyte: A relatively immature cell in the granulocyte series that is characterized by the presence of azurophilic (primary) granules.

Prorubricyte: Rubriblasts divide and differentiate into prorubricytes, which are somewhat smaller than rubriblasts, and which have slightly more condensed chromatin. Nucleoli are absent.

-R-

Rubriblasts: The most immature erythroid precursor that is morphologically recognizable in the bone marrow. It is characterized by a round nucleus with minimally condensed chromatin, a nucleolus, and intensely basophilic, agranular cytoplasm.

Rubricyte: Prorubricytes divide and differentiate into rubricytes, which are somewhat smaller than prorubricytes, and which have moderately condensed chromatin. The tinctorial quality of the cytoplasm depends on the concentration of hemoglobin.

-S-

Secondary granules: The granules that develop at the myelocyte stage of development of myeloid cells are used to identify granulocytes as neutrophils, eosinophils, or basophils.

Segmented neutrophil: The most terminally differentiated cell of the granulocyte series.

Spicule: A particle of bone marrow that is composed of adipocytes, hematopoietic cells, and the supportive connective tissue elements.

Stem cell factor: A pleiotropic cytokine with multiple systemic effects, one of which is to stimulate erythropoiesis.

Stem cell: Cells that have the capacity for self-renewal and the ability to differentiate along multiple cell lines (ie, pluripotential). All hematopoietic cells are derived from a common pluripotential stem cell.

Suggested Reading

Alleman AR, Harvey JW. The morphologic effects of vincristine sulfate on Canine Bone Marrow Cells. *Vet Clin Pathol*. 1993;22:36.

Bennett JM, et al. Proposals for the classification of the acute leukemias. *Brit J Haematol*. 1976;33:451.

Breuer W, et al. Bone-Marrow Changes in Infectious Diseases and Lymphohaemopoietic Neoplasms in Dogs and Cats—A Retrospective Study. *J Comp Pathol*. 1998;119:57.

Brown DE, et al. Cytology of Canine Malignant Histiocytosis. *Vet Clin Pathol*. 1994;23:118.

Brunning RD. Acute Myeloid Leukemias. Proceedings from the Annual Meeting of the American Society of Veterinary Clinical Pathologists.1985;135.

Carter RF, Valli VEO. Advances in the cytologic diagnosis of canine lymphoma. *Semin in Vet Med Surg Small Anim*. 1988;3:167.

Cowell RL, Tyler RD, Meinkoth JH. *Diagnostic Cytology and Hematology of the Dog and Cat*. 2nd ed. St. Louis, MO: Mosby; 1999.

Dale DC, et al. Long-term Treatment of Canine Cyclic Hematopoiesis with Recombinant Canine Stem Cell Factor. *Blood*. 1995;85:74.

Dellman HD, Eurell JA. *Textbook of Veterinary Histology*. 5th ed. Baltimore, MD: Williams & Wilkins; 1998.

Facklam NR, Kociba GJ. Cytochemical characterization of leukemic cells from 20 dogs. *Vet Pathol*. 1985;22:363.

Facklam NR, Kociba GJ. Cytochemical characterization of feline leukemic cells. *Vet Pathol*. 1986;23:155.

Fisher DJ, Naydan D, Werner LL, et al. Immunophenotyping lymphomas in dogs: A comparison of results from fine needle aspirate and needle biopsy samples. *Vet Clin Pathol*. 1995;24:118.

Greene CE. *Infectious Diseases of the Dog and Cat*. 2nd ed. Philadelphia, PA: WB Saunders; 1998.

Grindem CB, Perman VP, Stevens JB. Morphological classification and clinical and pathological characteristics of spontaneous leukemia in 10 cats. *J Amer Anim Hosp Assoc*. 1985;21:227.

Grindem CB, Stevens JB, Perman V. Cytochemical reactions in cells from leukemic dogs. *Vet Pathol*. 1986;23:103.

Grindem CB, Stevens JB, Perman V. Morphological classification and clinical and pathological characteristics of spontaneous leukemia in 17 dogs. *J Amer Anim Hosp Assoc*. 1985;21:219.

Henson KL, Alleman AR, Fox LE, et al. Diagnosis of disseminated adenocarcinoma by bone marrow aspiration in a dog with leukoerythroblastosis and fever of unknown origin. *Vet Clin Pathol*.1998;27:80.

Honeckman AL, et al. Diagnosis of Canine Immune-Mediated Hematologic Disease. *Comp Cont Ed*. 1996;18:113.

Jain NC, Blue JT, Grindem CB, et al. Proposed criteria for classification of acute myeloid leukemia in dogs and cats. *Vet Clin Pathol*. 1991;20:63.

Jain NC. Classification of myeloproliferative disorders in cats using criteria proposed by the Animal Leukaemia Study Group: A retrospective study of 181 cases (1969-1992). *Comp Haematol Int*. 1993;3:125.

Jain NC. *Essentials of Veterinary Hematology*. Philadelphia, PA: Lea & Febiger; 1993.

Jain NC. *Schalm's Veterinary Hematology*. 4th ed. Philadelphia, PA: Lea & Febiger; 1993.

Jolly RD, Walkley SU. Lysosomal Storage Diseases of Animals: An Essay in Comparative Pathology. *Vet Pathol*. 1997;34:527.

Leifer CE, Matus RE, Patnaik AK, MacEwen EG. Chronic myelogenous leukemia in the dog, *J Am Vet Med Assoc*. 1983;183:686.

Lewis DC, Meyer KM. Canine Idiopathic Thrombocytopenia Purpura. *J Vet Intern Med*. 1996;10:207.

Mackin AJ, et al. Effects of Vincristine and Prednisone on Platelet Numbers and Function in Clinically Normal Dogs. *Am J Vet Res*. 1995;56:100.

Messick J, Carothers M, Wellman M. Identification and characterization of megakaryoblasts in acute megakaryoblastic leukemia in a dog. *Vet Pathol*. 1990;27:212.

Pollet L, Van Hove W, Mathheeuws D. Blastic crisis in chronic myelogenous leukemia in a dog. *J Small Anim Prac*. 1978;19:469.

Quesenberry PJ. The concept of the hematopoietic stem cell. In: Hematology. 3rd ed. Williams WJ, Beutler E, Erslev AJ, Lichtman MA, eds. New York, NY: McGraw-Hill.

Raskin RE. Myelopoiesis and Myeloproliferative Disorders. *Vet Clin N Am Small Anim Prac*. 1996;26:1023.

Stokol T, Blue JT. Pure Red Cell Aplasia in Cats: 9 Cases (1989-1997). *J Am Vet Med Assoc*. 1999;214:75.

Swenson CL, et al. Cyclic Hematopoiesis Associated with Feline Leukemia Virus Infection in Two Cats. *J Am Vet Med Assoc*. 1987;191:93.

Vail DM, Moore AS, Ogilvie GK, et al. Feline lymphoma (145 cases): Proliferation indices, cluster of differentiation 3 immunoreactivity, and their association with prognosis in 90 cats. *J Vet Int Med*. 1998;12:349.

Walker D, Cowell RL, Clinkenbeard KD, et al. Bone marrow mast cell hyperplasia in dogs with aplastic anemia. *Vet Clin Pathol*. 1997;26:106-112.

Walton RM, et al. Bone Marrow Cytological Findings in 4 Dogs and a Cat with Hemophagocytic Syndrome. *J Vet Int Med*. 1996;10:7.

Wellman ML, Couto CG, Starkey RJ, Rojko JL. Lymphocytosis of large granular lymphocytes in three dogs. *Vet Pathol*. 1989;26:158.

Wellman ML, Davenport DJ, Morton D, Jacobs RM. Malignant histiocytosis in four dogs. *J Am Vet Med Assoc*. 1985;187:919.

Young NS, Maciejewski J. The Pathophysiology of Acquired Aplastic Anemia. *New Eng J Med*. 1997;336:1365.

Subject Index

Notes

Notes

Notes

Notes

Ralston Purina Company **Bone Marrow Evaluation in Dogs and Cats**